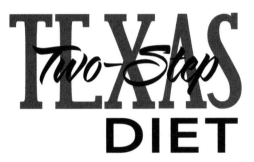

TEXAS *Two-Step* DIET

BRIGHT SKY PRESS

Box 416, Albany, Texas 76430

10   9   8   7   6   5   4   3   2   1

Library of Congress Cataloging-in-Publication Data

Bridgman, John C., 1937–
    Texas two-step diet : achieve happiness and health even when faced with cheese
  enchiladas / John C. Bridgman, Amy D. Bradshaw.
      p. cm.
    ISBN 1-931721-49-1 (alk. paper)
1. Weight loss. I. Bradshaw, Amy D., 1975– II. Title.

  RM222.2.B78134 2005
  613.2'5-dc22

2005041031

Book and cover design by Isabel Lasater Hernandez

Printed in China through Asia Pacific offset

John C. Bridgman
Amy D. Bradshaw, RD, LD

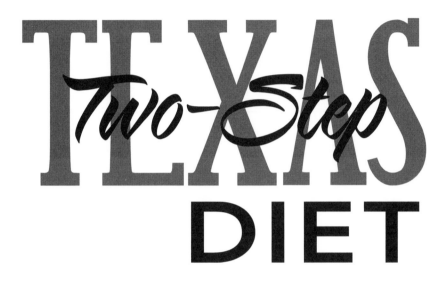

TEXAS
Two-Step
DIET

**Achieve happiness and health—
even when faced
with cheese enchiladas**

BRIGHT SKY PRESS

Albany, Texas

To my parents, who taught me to live these principles and be the best that I can be in life. I could never thank you enough!

To my husband, who supported me during the endless time I spent on my computer, working on this project.

And to John, who gave me this opportunity to share my passion in life with so many others.

—Amy Bradshaw

The top two priorities in my book *Time Out ... It's Your Call* are "Love" and "Family." These are the top two priorities in my life. I take this opportunity to express my appreciation to all my family for their support, love and understanding. I love you all very much!

And many thanks to Amy for her knowledgeable and practical contributions to the book. She is a great Texas Two-Step partner!

— John Bridgman

Contents

Get them enchiladas greasy.
Get them steaks chicken-fried.
Sho' do make a man feel happy
To see white gravy on the side.

—Guy Clark, "Texas Cookin'"

Don't blame Texas because you're fat. Whether or not you live here, if you're reading this book, you probably think like a Texan. You crank your SUV to drive two blocks. You love chili cheeseburgers, deep-fried catfish, and Blue Bell Cookies 'n Cream—and you like your helpings big. You order extra cream gravy with your chicken-fried steak, extra cheese in your enchiladas, and take an extra slice of pecan pie. It's not my fault, you think. Blame those ribs; blame the margaritas. The food made me do it.

Self-denial isn't part of the Texan psyche. But hope is, to a degree that's downright embarrassing. (Think Enron.) And if we told you that we'd found the diet secret you've been waiting for—the one that will melt your stubborn fat deposits even as you wolf down combination dinners—well, you'd buy that book, wouldn't you?

This isn't that book. The sad truth is that, even in Texas, quick fixes rarely lead to dramatic long-term improvements. The way to lose weight is, in fact, simple—but it's not easy or fast. The way to lose weight is to eat well and exercise. Plain as that.

But wait—don't put this book back on the shelf. You already know the basic ideas, but you haven't been putting them into practice, have you? That's where the *Texas Two-Step Diet* comes in. The dance we'll teach you involves determination and dedication—the two steps Texans (and anyone else) must take for health and happiness.

Determination, the first of the two steps, means mentally preparing yourself to succeed. You set priorities, deciding what is most important to you.

Whatever big dream you're chasing, you've got to refuse to let your weight hold you back.

Dedication, the crucial second step, is about following through on your goals, giving yourself the tools and help you need to succeed. William Barret Travis was clear on his priorities when he wrote, "God and Texas—Victory or Death!" But he and the other defenders of the Alamo needed reinforcements. And in both life and weight control, you'll need them, too. It's no fun to dance alone.

Doing the Texas Two-Step means going with the plan and making things happen. We offer sixteen action points to change your everyday life. Get on the beam with all sixteen, and you *will* lose weight. With determination and dedication, you'll keep it off. You'll look better, you'll feel better, and life will be loads more fun.

Doing what's right isn't the problem.
It's knowing what's right.

—Lyndon Baines Johnson

Chapter 1

Asking Questions

Do you want to achieve and maintain a healthy weight *or* do you want to live in an unfit, overweight body? It's not much of a question, is it? You don't want to be fat. You'd rather be thin, or at least thinner than you are today—ideally at your healthy weight. (In chapter 5, we'll demonstrate how to determine that weight.) By asking and answering that first question, you've already begun the Texas Two-Step.

So let's continue by asking a few more questions.

What?

- What will it take to succeed?
- What will I need to do?
- What advice do I need to follow?
- What am I trying to achieve?

Why?

- Why should I try this approach to losing weight?
- Why am I reading this book?
- Why do I think I will succeed this time?

When?

- When is the right time to start?
- When will I know it's working?
- When will I be successful?

How?

- How can I lose this weight?
- How can I maintain this weight loss?
- How can I enjoy social functions without feeling deprived?
- How can I have fun and lose weight at the same time?

Where?

- Where should I go for information?
- Where will I find the answers?

QUESTIONS AND ANSWERS

- Ask the right questions for the right reasons.
- Don't ask questions if you're not prepared for the answer.
- Don't answer a question if the person asking is not prepared for the answer.
- Not all questions require an answer. Be kind and considerate when asking or answering.
- Be a good listener. What is the real reason for the question?

Who?

- Who should I talk to?
- Who will join me in losing weight?
- Who will stick with me all the time?

Think about those questions. We'll come back to them in chapter 4.

Kick It Up!

Begin thinking of ways to kick up your whole family's diet … not just for weight loss, but with a healthier and more versatile menu.

Herb and vegetable gardening is very easy, inexpensive, interesting, decorative, delicious and good exercise for those working towards a healthier lifestyle. You can place herbs and even some vegetables among your landscape, flower beds or in pots, or you can make a small plot devoted just to your veggies and herbs.

Find herbs and vegetables that are suitable to your area. Most herbs and many vegetables are heat- and drought-tolerant, and some are even perennial.

Some of our favorite herbs:

Basil (Sweet, Lemon, Thai, Greek, small leaved, lettuce leaved, dwarf and tall)
Chives
Sage
Parsley (Curly or Italian flat leafed)
Lemon Balm
Oregano
Rosemary
Cilantro
Scented Geraniums
Mint (Spearmint, chocolate, peppermint, pineapple mint)
Thyme
Lavender

Some of our favorite vegetables for smaller spaces:

Lettuces
Salad Greens
Tomatoes (Cherry, grape, yellow pear, Super Sweet 100s, many heirloom varieties)
Peppers (Bell, sweet banana, hot banana, jalapeño, poblano, serrano)
Onion
Garlic

I shall never surrender or retreat.

—William Barret Travis,

letter from the Alamo

Chapter 2

Pros and Cons

Action Point One:
Sit right down and write yourself a letter

Why write a letter? Because writing is powerful. Writing will make your thoughts clearer and better organized, and when you're finished, you'll have something more than thoughts: You'll have a written record of them, which you can use to remind yourself of your goals.

In this letter, you should consider the pros and cons of losing weight, and make up your mind whether to commit to doing it. This letter is for you and you alone, so be honest.

As an example, here's a copy of John's letter to himself.

> *Dear John,*
>
> *I have been thinking about losing weight for a long time. I just don't seem to be motivated or committed enough to do it. I know I can lose weight if I really want to. So why don't I just do it? Why don't I get started? What am I waiting for? Why have I not been motivated enough?*
>
> *Here are my lists of the pros and cons of losing weight.*

Pros: Reasons why I should lose weight
• *The health payoff is huge—and it will be easier and more effective to lose the weight now than after I've begun suffering weight-related diseases such as heart disease or diabetes.*
• *I will feel better.*
• *I will look better.*
• *My clothes will fit better.*
• *I will have more energy.*
• *Carrying an extra 25 pounds is hard on my heart, my knees and many other parts of my body.*
• *Staying healthy means I will live longer to see my family grow.*
• *I will snore less.*
• *I will have less heartburn.*
• *I might improve my golf game.*
• *I will set a good example for others I care about.*
• *I won't make such a large splash when I dive into a pool.*
• *I will be able to keep up with my grandchildren better.*
• *I have tried before and failed. Succeeding this time would be all the sweeter.*
• *Just because it's the right thing to do, and I know it's time.*

Cons: Reasons why I shouldn't lose weight
• *I like to eat, drink and be merry.*
• *I won't have to buy a new wardrobe or alter my clothes.*
• *I am lazy.*
• *I procrastinate.*
• *Dieting might make me grouchy.*
• *It's hard work.*

It's obvious which list wins. I've got lots of good reasons to lose weight—and only weak ones to keep it on!

So what do I do, and how do I do it? I commit to finding the answers and following through.

Sincerely,
John

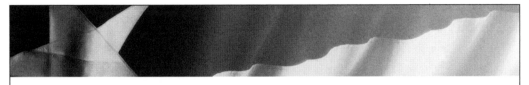

WRITE IT DOWN!

- Do the right things consistently, and in time you will get the right results.
- Keep a little notebook with you at all times.
- Take notes when you hear something you want to remember.
- Even for little decisions, make lists of pros and cons. Write down what you know and what you don't know.
- Take time to put your most important thoughts in writing.

After you have written yourself a personal and honest letter, read the letter again. Look at the three or four most striking reasons for losing weight and ask yourself, Are these enough? If they are important enough to motivate you (and they should be), then turn to the next chapter.

Alternative to Action Point One: Copy the list

Ask yourself whether you agree with these thoughts:
If I lose weight …

- I will feel better.
- I will look better and have better self-confidence.
- I will have more energy.
- I will live a longer, healthier life.

If you agree, copy that list and tape it to your bathroom mirror or your fridge—wherever it can remind you, several times a day, of your goals.

*Decide what you want, decide what you
are willing to exchange for it.
Establish your priorities and go to work.*
—Oil tycoon H.L. Hunt

Chapter 3

Priorities

Action Point Two:
List what's important to you

Texans take a businesslike approach to much of life—and weight loss is one area that could benefit. At many top companies, consultants talk about working *smarter,* not *harder.* They urge clarifying goals and priorities. They tell you to keep asking, "Are we making progress?"

What about You, Inc.? Are you working smart? What are your personal priorities? If you can't list them clearly, how can you expect to make the most of your life?

First, write down the top five priorities in your personal life today—the things you *really* want most to accomplish in your lifetime.

Next, write down the top five priorities in your work life. Same thing: What is it that you want most to do? Be honest.

Now, over the next week, make a record of how you spend your time. You can make your own time categories or use the ones below as a guide.

Personal

- Spending high-quality time with family
- Spending high-quality time with friends
- Watching television

- Eating
- Sleeping
- Reading
- Exercising
- Entertaining
- Enjoying movies, plays or concerts
- Doing housework
- Cooking
- Shopping
- Taking classes
- Working in the yard
- Paying bills, taking care of finances
- Attending athletic events
- Studying
- Playing computer games

Work

- Writing reports
- Attending meetings
- Reading and writing e-mail
- Talking on the phone
- Meeting with customers
- Handling complaints or problems
- Coaching
- Delegating
- Discussing budgets
- Doing strategic planning
- Traveling
- Reading
- Having lunch
- Training
- Making the company's product

Is there a difference between your five priorities and the way you spend your time? Should you consider making adjustments in your daily life?

Now ask yourself, Where does losing weight fit into my priorities? Even if you didn't list it—or list maintaining your physical and mental health—you almost certainly have goals that you won't accomplish unless you're healthy. To do what's important, you have to take care of yourself.

Consider how losing weight could affect your personal and business lives. How important to each of your priorities is feeling good, looking good, having more energy and self-confidence, and living a longer, healthier life?

What is really important to you in life? I think you know— and if you need a reminder why

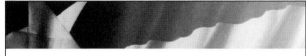

TAKE CONTROL OF YOUR TIME

- Say no sometimes. Your time is limited. Remember that if you say yes to one thing, you'll probably have to say no to something else.
- Do it now! That way you won't forget.
- Today promise yourself to eliminate two or three of your regular habits that are wastes of time. Put your commitment in writing.
- Decide to have a good, productive day today.
- Be conscientious about doing first things first.
- For more help setting your priorities, see John Bridgman's book *Time Out … It's Your Call.*

you need to lose weight, you need only pull out your list of priorities. Look at it frequently.

Alternative to Action Point Two: List Your Priorities

List the five things that matter most to you. Your list might look like this:
Family, health, happiness, church, success

Now ask yourself whether losing weight will help you in the areas that matter most.

*There are no problems that we cannot
solve together, and very few that we
can solve by ourselves.*

—Lyndon Baines Johnson

Chapter 4

Two-Step Partners

Action Point Three:
Ask for help

Texans are self-reliant, but we also understand that there are things a person doesn't do alone. One cowboy can't handle an entire cattle drive. Troy Aikman would have been nowhere without the rest of the Cowboys. And two-stepping alone looks silly.

Think of at least one person you like to spend time with, and who'll support your goal of losing weight and leading a healthier life. Maybe it's your spouse; maybe it's your neighbor; maybe it's your best friend. Whoever it is, that's your Texas Two-Step partner.

Tell your partner what you want to do, and that you're serious about it. Then ask for specific kinds of support. Those could include:

- Eating healthy meals with you.
- Exercising with you.
- Celebrating your successes (in a healthy way, of course).
- Simply asking, every day, how well you've stuck with your commitment.

If you're lucky, your partner wants to lead a healthier life, too. Then, of course, you can support each other.

Last, remember that even if your main dance partner is terrific, it's good to dance with other people, too. Enlist all the partners you can. Consider your kids, your boss, your parents, or your minister. If you can't find anyone to exercise with you, think about hiring a personal trainer or becoming a regular in an exercise class. If you're a regular at a restaurant, ask the waiter and the cook for their help.

You don't need to do this alone.

Answering the Questions

With your main Two-Step Partner, consider the answers to the questions we asked in chapter 1.

What?

- What will it take to succeed? *Dedication and determination.*
- What will I need to do? *Follow the action points.*
- What am I trying to achieve? *A healthier life.*

Why?

- Why should I try this approach to losing weight? *Because it's a real, long-term solution.*
- Why am I reading this book? *Because I'm ready to lose weight.*
- Why do I think I will succeed this time? *Because this time, I'm not on a fad diet. And this time, I have help.*

When?

- When is the right time to start? *Right now.*
- When will I know it's working? *When I feel healthier and look better.*
- When will I be successful? *I'm already succeeding—just by committing to my goal.*

How?

- How can I lose this weight? *By following all the action points in this book.*
- How can I maintain this weight loss? *By remembering that this isn't a diet. It's a long-term commitment, a new way of life.*

- How can I enjoy social functions without feeling deprived? *By remembering that social functions are just that: social. They're about people, not food. I'll try to focus on the people. (And I'll also use the tips in chapter 22.)*
- How can I have fun and lose weight at the same time? *By exercising and socializing with my Two-Step partners.*

Where?

- Where should I go for information? *This book is a good start—as are doctors, dietitians, and personal trainers.*
- Where will I find the willpower? *I've already begun to find it—through other people, and by committing to myself.*

Who?

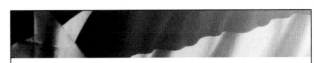

HELP AND BE HELPED

- Call an old friend today, just to say hello.
- Do something special for your spouse, a friend, or someone in your family.
- Do a little act of kindness for a stranger.
- Thank someone who you should have thanked before.
- Tell someone you're sorry for something you did in the past.
- Help someone—in the right way, for the right reason.
- Help someone anonymously.

- Who should I talk to? *My Two-Step partners.*
- Who will join me in losing weight? *My Two-Step partners.*
- Who will stick with me all the time? *My Two-Step partners.*

Supplemental Action Point

If you're a believer, turn to God. Who could possibly be in a better position to help?

Go through those questions from chapter 1—this time, considering God as one of your Two-Step partners.

Consider writing your own prayer or using this one:

Dear God,

I'm asking for your help because I haven't been able to do this alone before. Please give me the strength to avoid temptations. Help me all day long to do what I know must be done. Please keep me focused on my priorities so that I do not forget about my goals. And please guide my actions as I strive for those goals.

Help me throughout the day to have the strength and willpower to treat my body as you intended.

Amen

Basic Broth and Simple Soup

Basic Chicken Broth

Basic Broth can be a great partner for many dishes. You will always want to have some on hand. It is so delicious and so much more beneficial than the processed version.

Never throw away your chicken bones! Crack them and put them in a big stew pot with:

Water to cover
Onion
Celery
Carrots
Parsley
Bay leaves
Salt and freshly ground pepper to taste
(Get the picture? Use whatever flavors you love and whatever vegetables and herbs you have on hand.)

Heat to boiling and then let simmer for a couple of hours. Using a sieve, strain out the vegetables and bones and put broth back in the pot. You may season to your taste, but taste first. It may be just right!

You can then refrigerate or freeze the broth in containers for later use.

Simple Vegetable Soup

Simmer your favorite vegetables (carrots, tomatoes, asparagus, broccoli with peeled stems, potatoes or squash) in Basic Chicken Broth until very tender. Blend or process in batches; season with fresh herbs, salt and pepper. Fold in a little nonfat plain yogurt after blending for a creamier consistency. For a protein boost, toss in leftover chicken or ham.

A doctor asked an Aggie,
"How much do you weigh naked?"
The Aggie replied, "I don't know.
Without my glasses, I can't see the scale."

—Anonymous

Chapter 5

Finding What's Right for You

Action Point Four:
Analyze yourself

How Much Should You Weigh?

You want to be healthier and look better—but what does that mean? You wonder: What *should* I weigh? What is my healthy weight? What should I aim for? The answer: It depends.

Your healthy weight may not match the recommendation of the height-and-weight charts. Those numbers are approximate, but one size doesn't fit all. You need to figure out the weight that's best for you.

Your body already knows this weight. It's your pre-established "set point," the weight that you naturally maintain when you're leading a healthy life, eating right and exercising regularly.

Your *Approximate* Healthy Weight

Let's begin by making a rough estimate of your healthy weight.

For men: Start with 106 and add an additional six pounds for every inch of your height over five feet. This number is the low end of your healthy weight range.

To get the high end, add an additional 10 percent.

For example, if you're six foot two, your calculations would look like this:

Low end: 106 + (6 × 14)=190
High end: 190 + (190 × 0.10)=209

So if you're six-foot-two-inch man, you should weigh between 190 and 209 pounds.

For women: To get the low end of your healthy weight range, start with 100 and add an additional five pounds for every inch of your height over five feet. To get the high end, take that number and add 10 percent.

If you're five foot four, your calculations would look like this:

Low end: 100 + (5 × 4)=120
High end: 120 + (120 × 0.10)=132

So if you're a five-foot-four-inch woman, your healthy weight range would be between 120 and 132 pounds.

Your Body Mass Index

Body mass index (BMI) is another means of relating your weight to your height. To calculate your BMI:

1. Multiply your weight in pounds by 0.45
   For example: 140 pounds × 0.45=63

2. Multiply your height in inches by 0.025 and then square the answer (Remember, there are 12 inches in a foot).
   For example, if you're five foot ten (70 inches), you'd calculate:
   (70 × 0.025) × (1.75 × 1.75)=3.06

3. Take your answer from 1), and divide it by your answer in 2).
   63 ÷ 3.06=20.59

4. Compare your number to BMI scales.

A BMI from 18.5 to 24.9 is considered healthy.
A BMI from 25 to 30 is considered overweight.
A BMI greater than 30 is considered obese.

In our example, a person with a BMI of 20.59 would be at a healthy weight.

Percentage Body Fat

Of course, it's not just your total weight that matters, or even your weight adjusted for your height. What matters is how much of your body is fat.

The BMI assumes that you have a standard amount of muscle, and if that's not true, the BMI range won't be right for you. Because muscle weighs much more than fat, a muscular weight lifter may weigh more than his BMI range recommends—even though he doesn't need to lose an ounce. On the other hand, a person who's lost muscle mass because of aging, sickness or extreme inactivity may be carrying too much fat, even though his BMI falls within the healthy range.

If you think you fall into either of those categories—or if you're just curious—you'll want to hire a professional to measure your percentage body fat. He or she will use calipers or a bioimpedence machine—or, most accurate of all, hydrostatic weighing.

Other Factors

In setting your weight goal, you also need to consider these things:

- **Your age.** As you get older, you naturally lose muscle, your metabolism naturally slows down, and the pounds tend to stay on.
- **Your diet history.** The more diets you have attempted in the past, the more likely it is that you have lowered your metabolism enough to decrease your calorie needs. Crash dieting also can change your body composition. When you lose weight, you lose water, fat and muscle. When you regain the weight, you gain mainly fat and water. Therefore, you have just changed your body composition for the worse by increasing your body fat percentage.
- **Your physical activity.** You need regular exercise, not only to burn calories, but also to improve your body composition. A pound of muscle burns more calories,

even when you're not using it, than a pound of fat. So the more muscle you have, the faster your metabolism—and the easier it is to keep off the pounds.

- **Your body shape.** Are you shaped like an apple or a pear? Apples are round, storing fat in their abdomens or upper bodies. Pears store it down below, in their hips, buttocks and thighs. In general, it's better to be a pear than an apple. As your waist expands, your health risks climb. People with fat concentrated in their upper bodies show increased risk of health concerns such as diabetes, heart disease, and high blood pressure. This is especially true if a man's waist is more than 40 inches, or a woman's is more than 35.

To determine your risk, calculate your waist-to-hip ratio. Measure your waist at its smallest point, and your hips at their largest point. (Don't cheat by wrapping the tape too tight.) Then divide your waist measurement by your hip measurement. A man's waist-to-hip ratio should be 0.95 or lower. A woman's should be 0.80 or lower.

Setting Your Goal

Answer each of the following questions honestly, then use the analysis that follows to set your healthy weight goal.

1. What is your approximate healthy weight?
2. What is your BMI?
3. Is your BMI within the healthy-weight range (18.5 to 24.9)?
4. If your BMI is not within the healthy range, at what weight would it be in the healthy range?
5. What is your body fat percentage?
6. What is your body shape (apple or pear)?
7. What is your waist-to-hip ratio?
8. On a scale of one to ten (ten being the highest) how motivated are you at this time in your life to make the necessary changes?
9. At this time in your life, how much time can you realistically dedicate to exercise?
10. Is there a history of excess weight in your family (parents, grandparents, siblings)?
11. What is the lowest weight you have maintained for at least one year? How long did you stay at that weight?
12. What is your personal highest weight? How long did you stay at that weight?

Analyzing Your Answers

- If your answers to questions 1 through 7 suggest that losing weight would benefit your health, then losing weight should be one of your top priorities. If your BMI is greater than 25, your initial goal should be to lose 10 percent of your current weight.

  For example, a woman who is five foot six and weighs 175 pounds has a BMI of 29. Her initial weight-loss goal would be 10 percent of her current weight (175 × .10=17.5 pounds). And if she lost that 17.5 pounds, she'd weigh 157.5 pounds.

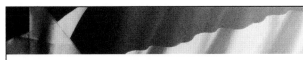

THE PLAIN TRUTH ABOUT LOSING WEIGHT

- To shed pounds, you either need to consume fewer calories than you normally burn, or through extra exercise, burn more calories than you normally consume. Or, best of all, do both.

- No matter what the source of your calories—carbohydrates, proteins or fats—when you consume more than you burn, they will be stored as body fat.

- Question 8 measures your dedication and determination—the steps in the Texas Two-Step. If you scored yourself 7 or higher, great! But if you scored lower than 7, ask yourself why you're not more motivated. (Are you unsure whether you can make changes? Have tried and failed in the past? Do you have no support?) Use this book's action points to address those problems.

- If your answer to question 9 was "none," you need to reassess your priorities. Exercise is crucial to your health, and it's impossible to maintain long-term weight loss without it. Any exercise at all is enough to start.

- If you answered "yes" to question 10, your family history of obesity suggests that you need to use an "adjusted body weight."
  (For more information, see the box "Calculating Your Adjusted Body Weight.")

- Question 11 asked about the lowest weight you've maintained for a year. If you have been at your lowest weight within the last two years, you may be able to achieve this weight again. The longer you've carried extra pounds, the harder it is to shed them.

- If you have been at your highest weight or close to it for the last five years or more, you too should use an "adjusted body weight" as your goal.

How much should you eat?

Now that you have determined your healthy weight, it's time to figure out how to reach it. How much you should eat each day?

The answer, once again, is: It depends.

Age, gender, genetics, and body composition all affect your metabolism. The more muscle you have, the higher your metabolism will be. Even while resting, a muscular person burns more calories than a person without much muscle.

Let's begin by calculating your resting metabolic rate (RMR) adjusted for your healthy weight. Your RMR is the number of calories your body burns while hardly moving—say, while you're in bed. It's the energy you need just to survive: to breathe and to pump your blood. For most of us, those most basic activities require about 60 percent of the calories we burn each day.

Digesting food takes up another 10 percent of your day's calories. (Yes, it actually costs you calories to eat!)

But, of course, eating and sleeping isn't all you do. Maybe you walk, jog, ride horseback, do yoga, or garden. Maybe you chase toddlers around the house. Even relatively sedentary people run errands, do housework, and walk from their desks to the coffee maker. And those activities burn your remaining allotment of calories for the day.

When calculating what you need, we call the calories you burn through action "the activity factor." That's the tricky part of the calculation, and a professional dietician or personal trainer can help you calculate your exact needs and tailor a plan precisely to you.

We also need to keep your age in mind. In adulthood, your energy needs decline approximately 2 percent per decade. This is due to changes in hormones and body composition. As you age, unless you exercise regularly, you lose muscle mass—and without those muscles, you burn fewer calories, even at rest.

Calculating Your Adjusted Body Weight

Let's face it: If you're significantly overweight or have a family history of obesity, you'll have a harder time reaching your healthy weight. It's important that you make your goal a personal healthy weight that you can achieve and maintain. Keep your priorities straight: You want to improve your health, not be super-model-thin. Remember, fit, fabulous, gorgeous people come in *all* sizes.

The good news is that even if you're obese, if you can maintain a 10 percent weight loss, your health will improve dramatically. Resolve not just to lose the weight, but to keep it off. Yo-yo dieting is harder on your health than not losing weight in the first place.

But what should your goal be? To figure your adjusted body weight, take your current weight and subtract from it the lower number of your approximate healthy weight figured earlier.

For example, consider a five-foot-six woman who weighs 175 pounds. Her approximate healthy weight range is 130 to 136.5 pounds.
175–130=45

Multiply your result by 0.25
45 × 0.25=11.25

To get your goal range, add your answer to both the lower and the higher number of your approximate healthy weight range.
130 + 11.25=141
136.5 + 11.25=148

This woman should aim to weigh between 141 and 148 pounds.

1. Calculate your RMR, adjusted for your new healthy weight goals:

    Women: Multiply your "healthy weight" by 10.
    Men: Multiply your "healthy weight" by 11.

2. Add some calories for your daily activities. Choose the activity level that best describes you. (And yes, you have to be honest.)

- Activity factor of 1.2
  You're not very active. You don't have an exercise routine. You look for the closest parking spot and always choose the elevator instead of the stairs. You spend your day behind a desk, in front of the television or doing a few light chores. (If this is you, turn next to the exercise chapter. We don't have a day to lose.)

- Activity factor of 1.3
  You don't have any specific exercise, but you're up and about during the day— busy taking care of children, walking dogs, doing chores or moving around at work.

- Activity factor of 1.4
  You exercise, but you don't worry about getting it in every single day. You'd rather walk the dogs than watch TV at night, and your many responsibilities keep you busy, up and about.

- Activity factor of 1.5
  Stop and pat yourself on the back. Kudos to you, kid! You have a regular exercise program, with aerobic activity at least five days a week. You're probably fidgety, willing to take the stairs. If there's not a close spot in the parking lot, it doesn't bother you in the least to walk.

Multiply your RMR by your activity factor. The answer is the number of calories you need to consume each day to maintain your *current* weight.

3. Calculate how much you need to adjust your daily intake.
   To lose weight:

- To lose ten pounds or less, subtract 200 calories.
- To lose between eleven and twenty-five pounds, subtract 300 calories.
- To lose more than twenty-five pounds, subtract 500 calories.

To gain weight:

- To gain ten pounds, add 200 calories.
- To gain eleven to twenty-five pounds, add 400 calories.

1. A 53-year-old male who is six feet tall and has weighed 175 the majority of his life (his personal set point). But in the last six months, after a job crisis became overwhelming, he gained twenty pounds. He became much more sedentary. Though he'd once trained for marathons, now he felt lucky to get his thirty-minute jogs twice a week. Still, he wants to lose those twenty pounds.

   To get his RMR, we multiply his healthy weight times the factor for men:
   175 × 11=1925

   Then, to calculate his total calorie needs for the day at his *current* weight, we multiply his RMR by his activity factor—his current activity factor, not his old one:
   1925 × 1.3=2503

   To figure out how much he should eat to lose twenty pounds, we subtract 300:
   2503–300=2203

2. A 29-year-old female is five-foot-ten and very active. She has weighed around 140 pounds for approximately five years now. She bikes five or six times a week and does weight training twice a week. She wants to maintain her weight.

   To calculate her RMR, we multiply her healthy weight (140) times the factor for women:
   140 × 10=1400

   Then, to calculate her calorie needs to maintain her current rate, we multiply her RMR by her activity level:
   1400 × 1.5=2100

Note: It's important that you do consume at least 1200 calories per day, no matter what your calculations show.

Alternative to Action Point Four:
Hire a pro

Hire a personal trainer or a dietician, and let the pro crunch the numbers for you. The alternative is especially recommended if you're a special case—if you're obese, if you have health problems, if you're especially muscular, or if you're especially lacking in muscle. A pro knows how to handle all those circumstances.

Dress to Impress!

Processed salad dressings are a big no-no! They are full of sugars, additives, preservatives and salt. The best way to enhance the flavor of your foods is by dressing it up with homemade dressings and salsas. This will ensure that you are benefiting from the fresh herbs and vegetables and not loading up on the extra calories and non-natural ingredients.

Cilantro-Jalapeño Dressing

1 bunch cilantro (1 cup leaves)
2 cloves minced garlic
1 jalapeño, seeded (more if you desire more hotness)
¼ cup white wine vinegar
¼ cup water
½ tsp. salt
2 cups Easiest and Best Mayonnaise (without the herbs)

Puree all but mayonnaise in processor or blender. Fold mixture into mayonnaise. Chill two hours.

This is not only a great salad dressing but is wonderful spread on sandwiches and as a dip.

Vinaigrette

⅓ cup cider or wine vinegar
½–1 T. Dijon mustard
⅔ cup olive oil
½ tsp. sugar (optional)
Salt and pepper to taste
Chopped fresh herbs to taste

Combine all ingredients in a 12-ounce jar. Shake vigorously to combine. Correct seasonings to taste.

Note: Make "Lemonette" dressing by substituting fresh lemon juice for the vinegar. For more salad ideas, see page 44.

You really can eat more and weigh less—
if you know what to eat.

—Dean Ornish

Chapter 6

Foods for Health and Healing

Action Point Five:
Make your shopping list

With all the talk of decoding the human genome, you might think that your genes play the largest role in determining your overall health—so really, there's not much you can do to change your fate. This is not—repeat, *not*—the case.

According to Bradley Willcox, a Harvard Medical School researcher, genes account for only one-third of longevity. Willcox and two other researchers (D. Craig Willcox and Makoto Suzuki) spent 25 years studying the longest-lived people on earth: residents of Okinawa, a string of tropical islands between Japan and Taiwan. Okinawans routinely live into their nineties and beyond—and remain healthy and active at those older ages. Americans can only envy Okinawans' low rates of obesity, memory loss, heart disease, osteoporosis, and breast, colon and prostate cancer.

So what's the secret? After studying the islands' 100-year-olds, the researchers concluded that it was the Okinawans' lifestyle. The centenarians exercised, ate a low-fat diet, were careful about stress management, nurtured strong social and family ties, and felt spiritually connected. As younger Okinawans began adopting a less healthful lifestyle, their life expectancies dropped.

The bad news is that their less healthy lifestyle is ours—the modern Western lifestyle, complete with super-sized meals at the drive-through window.

The good news is we can change. Willcox writes that most of us have genes that will allow us to live into our eighties and nineties, but only if we adopt healthy habits.

Exercise and eating well are the most basic of those healthy habits. In this chapter, we'll focus on food—not the foods that you shouldn't eat, but the foods that you *should* eat.

"Powerhouse foods" are the ones most beneficial to your health.

Antioxidants: Health Powerhouses

When our bodies burn oxygen for energy, they produce an unpleasant byproduct: free radicals, molecules that yearn to capture an electron from some other molecule. Free radicals travel throughout the body, and as they capture those electrons from other molecules, they damage cells and create more free radicals. This damage can cause or contribute to disease.

You can't stop your body from creating free radicals, but by eating the right foods, you can neutralize them. Antioxidants are molecules that can donate an electron to a free radical without becoming free radicals themselves. They roam the body, fighting cell damage. In this way, antioxidants improve immune function and help lower the risk for cancer, heart disease, strokes, and cataracts. They're also believed to help slow aging.

The strongest evidence for antioxidant power lies with vitamins C, E, and beta carotene (which the body converts to vitamin A). To boost your antioxidants, be sure to eat foods that are rich in them.

- **For vitamin C:** citrus fruits, strawberries, kiwi, cantaloupe, green peppers, cabbage, spinach, kale and broccoli.

- **For vitamin E:** nuts, seeds, whole grains, vegetable and fish oils, fortified cereals and dried apricots.

- **For vitamin A:** spinach, carrots, squash, broccoli, yams, tomatoes, cantaloupe, peaches, fortified milk, and fortified grain products.

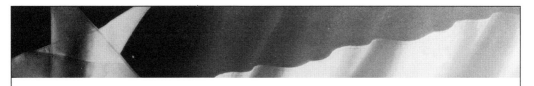

FOODS YOU CAN USE

- The anthocyanins found in red grapes, blueberries and strawberries may help us ward off heart disease by preventing clot formation. Add blueberries to your oat bran, grapes to your salad, and strawberries to your smoothie.
- The onion family is rich in allyl sulfides, which help lower blood pressure and protect against some cancers. Keep a bag of frozen chopped onions on hand, and add them to anything that strikes your fancy.
- Broccoli, cabbage and kale contain isothiocyanates that stimulate the liver to break down pesticides and carcinogens. Throw broccoli in your stir-fry, cabbage in your soup, and kale in your salad. Or use kale in any way that you'd use spinach.
- Sprinkle ground flaxseed on your high-fiber cereal, yogurt, salad or smoothie, for additional fiber and omega-3s.
- For healthy complex carbohydrates, try unusual grains such as quinoa, millet, amaranth, couscous and buckwheat.
- Look for ways to add more vegetables to daily meals. Add steamed zucchini, carrots, broccoli, and bell peppers to pasta dishes. Add tomato, cucumber, sprouts, and peppers to sandwiches. Sandwiches are also great with sliced pineapple, apple, and raisins. Stuff an omelette with veggies.
- Substitute wheat flour for half the white flour in baking recipes.

Functional Foods

We've already discussed how our bodies need energy (calories) to sustain life and carry out activities. "Functional foods" provide more than calories. They also enhance our health and protect us from disease.

Here are some of our favorites—foods that you ought to eat more of:

Fruits and vegetables are powerful in many ways. They provide vitamins, fiber, phytonutrients, and antioxidants. They're low in calories, and they help prevent cancer. Increasing your fruit and vegetable consumption is one of the most powerful ways you can improve your health.

Oats help lower cholesterol levels, and help maintain cholesterol levels that are already healthy.

Fatty fish, such as tuna, mackerel, salmon and sardines, contain omega-3 fatty acids, which lower your risk for heart disease and help improve mental performance. The American Heart Association recommends that people without heart disease eat fatty fish twice a week. People *with* heart disease should eat it even more often, or consider a supplement.

Yogurt contains live bacteria called lactobacillus. Lactobacillus lives naturally in the human gut, where it helps keep other bacteria in check.

Soy fights "bad" cholesterol. The American Heart Association says that eating 25 to 50 grams per day has been shown to lower blood levels of low-density lipids (or LDLs).

Green and black teas are antioxidants, which help protect from free radicals. (See the box "Antioxidants.")

Whole grains—to make the best-quality choices with your grains, simply remember, fiber, fiber, and more fiber! Choose wholesome, high-fiber carbs instead of refined, white-flour and high-sugar ones. At first, change all your breads to wheat or whole-grain. Eat wheat or rye crackers instead of saltines, sweet potatoes instead of white potatoes, brown or wild rice instead of white rice, whole-wheat pasta instead of regular pasta. And

42

obviously, you should choose high-fiber cereals instead of sugary kids' stuff. Bran flakes or Cocoa Puffs? That's a no-brainer.

Phytonutrients: Why a Carrot Beats a Multivitamin

To protect themselves from viruses, bacteria, and fungi, plants naturally produce substances called "phytonutrients" (or sometimes "phytochemicals"). Fruits and vegetables are full of phytonutrients. They provide color, aroma, flavor—and significant health benefits.

Scientists have identified several hundred phytonutrients, and they continue to discover more all the time. (Maybe you've heard about beta carotene, lutein, lycopene, and polyphenols.) According to the U.S. Department of Agriculture, phytonutrients can do your body a world of good: It's believed that they serve as antioxidants, enhance the immune response, help cell-to-cell communication, cause cancer cells to die, repair DNA damage caused by cigarette smoke and other toxins, and detoxify carcinogens.

The best way to consume your phytonutrients? Forget supplement pills or capsules, which may or may not provide health benefits. One study even shows that beta carotene supplements may *increase* smokers' chances of cancer. Scientists believe that to fight the large numbers of free radicals caused by smoking, beta carotene needs to work in concert with other nutrients, such as vitamins C and E, plus other antioxidant phytonutrients that may yet be undiscovered. Those healthful combinations occur naturally in food: Supplement makers can only dream of matching the powers of spinach or grapefruit.

Making Your List

Take out the pad that you normally use for your shopping list. First, write a list of five powerhouse foods that you can commit to using every week. Second, write a list of three powerhouse foods that you haven't eaten in a long time, but agree to try within the next week.

Take those two lists to the grocery store with you. Then tape those lists to the fridge, where you can glance at them every time you think about eating.

Alternative to Action Point Five:
Hire a dietitian to prepare a weekly menu for you.

Healing Power

So many vegetables and herbs have healing and medicinal qualities—and better to take your medicine in its pure form than in a little pill. Adding nuts to your salad gives it a super protein boost, and they are a healthy monounsaturated fat that helps you stay full longer.

Spinach and Strawberry Salad with Jicama Stars Salad

6 oz. fresh baby spinach
4 cups fresh strawberries, sliced
Jicama, peeled, sliced and cut into desired shape with cookie cutter
½ cup pecans. When time permits, toast pecans on cookie sheet in 300° oven for
    15 minutes. Keep an eye on them, so they don't get too toasty.

Dressing

½ cup canola oil
¼ cup white vinegar
2 T. sugar
1 T. poppy seeds
¼ tsp. paprika
¼ tsp. salt

Whisk dressing ingredients together in bowl. Pour over salad. Toss and serve. When strawberries are not in season, you can use other berries, cherries or oranges.

Romaine with Pears, Pecans and Feta

One head of romaine, rinsed well and torn into bite size pieces
2 firm ripe pears, peeled and thinly sliced
¼–½ cup fresh pecans, coarsely chopped or broken into pieces, or your favorite nut
4 ounces reduced-fat feta cheese
2 sprigs of fresh mint (optional)

Peel and thinly slice pears, and quickly pour a little Vinaigrette or Lemonette dressing (see page 37) over slices. Place romaine in salad bowl, and attractively arrange pears, pecans and crumbled feta cheese over top. Drizzle with more dressing. Scissor-cut mint leaves over the top. Toss. Serves 6–8.

Black Bean and Corn Salad

2 ears fresh corn, lightly cooked and removed from cob (or if you're desperate,
    1 can whole kernel corn, drained)
2 cups black or pinto beans, drained (either leftover or if desperate, canned)
4 large tomatoes, chopped
1 avocado, diced
4 green onions
1 large jalapeño, seeded and chopped
⅓ cup cilantro
¼ cup lime juice
2 tsp. ground cumin
½ tsp. salt
½ tsp. pepper
2 T. olive oil

Combine all ingredients.
This is another that can be altered to fit whatever you have in the garden or refrigerator.

Setting a goal is not the main thing.
It is deciding how you will go about
achieving it and staying with that plan.

—Tom Landry

Chapter 7

Don't Pull That Trigger!

Action Point Six:
Recognize your trigger points—and hold your fire

Amy often tells her clients to follow the 80–20 rule. Eighty percent of the time, you should make the best food choices possible, picking high-quality items that will best meet your nutritional needs. Twenty percent of the time, you can yield to your pleasure cravings, even if the foods aren't good for you.

Most of the time, the 80–20 rule is surprisingly easy to follow. You don't have to count calories; you just count choices. The 80–20 rule allows you to satisfy your hunger and still eat the foods you love. But the rule doesn't address the other reasons we eat.

Those reasons are emotional, and they're tough to address. Most of us don't eat only because we're hungry. Sometimes we eat because we're bored, or upset, or disappointed. We use food for comfort. We let it fill a void. But its solace is short-lived at best—and destructive at worst. A quart of Blue Bell Rocky Road won't fix a broken heart or transform your boss into a reasonable human being. But if you eat that quart every evening, it'll definitely change your body.

We don't overeat only when we're alone, of course. Maybe you take double servings of your mom's banana pudding every Sunday because it makes her smile. Or maybe you meet the same co-worker every Thursday for happy-hour nachos, margaritas, and complaints about the boss. A gigantic drink and vat of popcorn always enhances your weekly movie date with your spouse. How, you wonder, could anyone enter a baseball stadium without buying a chili dog and a giant beer? And what's a party without seven-layer dip and a few Shiner Bocks?

As if life weren't difficult enough, Texas restaurants specialize in temptation. Zagat restaurant surveys have shown that people in Houston and Dallas dine out more frequently than even New Yorkers. Restaurant food is often far less healthy than what you'd cook at home. The pitfalls of chicken-fried anything are obvious, but in restaurants, even grilled meats can be loaded with fat and salt. The portions are often twice the healthy size for a normal person—sometimes even bigger. And then, of course, there's the issue of dessert. If your dinner companion orders the death-by-chocolate cake, isn't it only polite to do the same?

Well, no. It's time to change your habits.

Stop now and think about your usual week. Ask yourself when it is that you blow the 80–20 rule. Then ask yourself *why* you do it.

Now, imagine strategies to handle those events and emotions in a way that won't wreck your body. Maybe you're overeating instead of addressing a big problem in your life: deep, day-to-day loneliness; a job you can't stand; a marriage on the rocks. If your problem is of that scale, resolve to address it head-on. If you don't know how to change what's making you miserable, talk with your friends, your family, or a professional counselor or minister. And while you're straightening out your life, remind yourself that an afternoon candy bar won't really make you happy.

Most of us, though, don't need a large-scale reason to overeat. And we can learn new ways to deal with the little stresses of everyday life.

For instance, if you find yourself noshing because you're bored, try devoting yourself to a new hobby. Learn to knit. Take up carpentry. Join a community garden. Volunteer to tutor a kid at a nearby school. Sign up for line-dancing classes. Go to your local bookstore and ask the most sympathetic-looking clerk to recommend a great, absorbing novel. Or better still: Sign up for an exercise class that meets every day.

Are you lonely sometimes? Call your Two-Step Partner, your mom, or an old friend. Track down your old college roommate or that friend you meant never to lose touch with. Join a volunteer group, a softball team, or a club that piques your interest. Look for an appealing Internet community. Or adopt a pet. (Dogs are especially good because they require walks; they're like furry exercise buddies. Besides, at dog parks, you meet other dog people.)

Stressed? Take a walk. Meditate or pray. Soak in a hot bath. Move your furniture around. Listen to music. Plan your next vacation. Get a massage. Or exercise: Working up a sweat really will melt your tension.

Are restaurants and social events your downfall? First of all, avoid temptations when you can. Consider meeting your friends someplace less fattening than usual. Instead of a restaurant rendezvous, you could take a walk together, go for a hike, go shopping, or play racquetball.

But of course you can't just avoid temptation. (We'll talk more about temptation in chapter 21.) The important thing is that when you find yourself tempted, you have a plan in place. Go ahead and go to the ball game—but eat at home first, or at least plan ahead what you'll order at the stadium. Discuss your weekly movie date with your spouse, and together you can eat a reasonable meal first and agree to bypass the snack counter. With your strategy in place, the oily popcorn and oversize Hershey bars won't seem half as alluring.

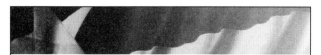

Contribute healthy food to social gatherings. A box of clementines, a fruit salad, a tray of veggies and dip, or a bowl of toasted cashews would be welcome at any party.

Remember, too, that it *is* possible to eat a healthy meal at a restaurant. A sub (with no cheese) makes a more satisfying lunch than a burger, and it's far better for you. Propose meeting at restaurants that serve healthy meals: soups, salads, lean meats and lots of vegetables. And if somehow you can't go to a place that doesn't ooze temptation, keep in mind that even McDonald's now offers salads, and most fast-food outlets are actively adding new healthy foods to their menus.

And if, in the end, you know it's not possible for you to resist a favorite restaurant dish—if sometimes you require fried shrimp to restore your soul—restrict that beloved dish to special occasions that fall under the 80–20 rule. A lot of good behavior leaves you room for a little indulgence.

Alternative to Action Point Six

We strongly recommend that you pursue Action Point Six. For most of us, understanding our trigger points and planning how to handle them is crucial to long-term success.

But if you think you're in the minority—that you can tough it out and simply resist temptations of social and emotional eating—see chapter 22 for more on developing your willpower.

Soup's On!

Soups can be your best friend. They are packed with nutritious vegetables, delicious herbs and are a great comfort food.

Roasted Red Bell Pepper Soup

2 large red bell peppers
1 tsp. olive oil
1 cup chopped onion
1 tsp. Chinese 5-Spice Powder
2 cloves garlic, minced
1 fresh tomato, diced (or ½ cup of tomato paste and ¼ cup of water)
¼ tsp. salt
⅛ tsp. black pepper
3 cups Basic Chicken Broth (see page 25)
Plain nonfat yogurt

Cut bell peppers in half lengthwise; discard seeds and membranes. Place peppers, skin side up, on a baking sheet; flatten with palm of hand. Broil peppers 3 inches from heat 10 minutes or until blackened and charred. Place peppers in ice water, and chill 5 minutes. Drain peppers; peel and discard skins. Set peppers aside.

Heat oil in large saucepan over medium heat. Add onion, Chinese 5-Spice Powder, and garlic; sauté 5 minutes. Add pepper, tomato and next 4 ingredients; stir well. Bring to a boil; cover, reduce heat and simmer 10 minutes.

Spoon mixture into blender (not all at once—it will splatter and burn you); cover and process until smooth.

Ladle into bowls; top with yogurt and garnish with a sprig of fresh parsley, cilantro or basil.

Whole Grains for a Whole Body

We grew up in a white bread world. Finally, there are many choices on the grocery shelves that offer whole grains in our breads, cereals, pastas and rices. Choose the whole grains—they do not taste much different, and they add that much needed fiber!

Watt's Wonder Muffs

2 cups whole-wheat flour
½ cup wheat germ
½ cup oat bran or 1 cup bran flakes, bran buds, or raisin bran
1 tsp. baking powder
1 tsp. baking soda
1 tsp. cinnamon
1 tsp. salt
¼ cup honey *or* ½ cup sugar
⅓ cup Canola oil
1 egg and 2 egg whites
2 tsp. vanilla

Preheat oven to 375°. Mix dry ingredients. Add honey or sugar, oil, eggs, vanilla, mix well. Add remaining ingredients.

Pour batter into lightly greased muffin cups or baking cups. Bake 25–30 minutes, or until toothpick inserted into center comes out clean.

Makes 24 muffins.

To add some zip, include 1 cup chopped apple, peach or pear; 2 plums, unpeeled; 1½ cups mashed banana (3 ripe); ½ cup raisins; or ½ cup pecans or walnuts.

Official state vegetable of Texas: 1015 Onion
Official state fruit: Texas red grapefruit

Chapter 8

Top Food Choices

In a state once ruled by oil, we take fuel seriously. And when it comes to fueling our bodies, quality matters as much as quantity. You wouldn't put oil in your gas tank and expect it to perform well, would you? In the same sense, you cannot fuel your body with junk and expect it to run properly. You need to make high-quality food choices the majority of the time.

Below we list high-quality foods that you should eat, foods that should serve as the foundation of your everyday meals and snacks. You'll be glad to see that the list is long—with lots of choices, lots of variety. Even so, it doesn't include every possible good choice. But you'll get the idea.

Wholesome Grains

Forget what you've heard in the last few years: Carbohydrates aren't evil. Think about the people you know who have always been thin, those who seem to have no problem maintaining a healthy weight. Do they eat carbs? Of course they do. Carbohydrates are your body's main source of fuel, and they serve as the foundation of any healthy long-term food plan.

But most likely your effortlessly thin friends aren't filling up on Twinkies, saltines, sugary cereals, and white bread. It's important to choose good carbohydrates—complex ones, which are digested slowly and don't wreak havoc on your blood sugar; high-fiber ones, which improve your digestion by acting as nature's broom; and, of course, those that include lots of vitamins and other nutrients.

Whole grains are a terrific source of carbohydrates. When grains are processed, up to 80 percent of their nutrients may be destroyed. But whole grains contain the entire kernel: the bran, or outer shell (full of B vitamins and fiber); the germ, or embryonic center (minerals, B vitamins, protein, vitamin E, and oils); and the endosperm between the kernel and the germ (starch, some protein). Even enriched flours are a poor substitute for whole grains because enrichment replaces only a few of the lost nutrients.

Try to eat a wide assortment of grains. Not only will you consume a greater variety of nutrients, but your food will be more interesting. In particular, try exploring some of the "new" grains on your grocery store's health-food shelf. Many are actually older than the Alamo; for centuries, they've served as staples around the world.

A few of our favorites:

Amaranth is really a seed rather than a proper cereal grain. It's rich in protein and, unlike other grains, supplies a good amount of calcium. For breakfast, try simmering amaranth along with another grain in a small amount of apple juice, then serve with yogurt and fresh fruit. For dinner, stir-fry amaranth with garlic, onion, and peppers. It's also a nice thickener for soups; add it during the last half-hour of cooking.

Barley, one of the first cultivated crops, has been used for food, medicine, and even a form of currency since biblical times. Most of the barley sold in the United States has been milled to remove the bran, but it's possible to find less-refined forms ("flakes," "grits," or "hulled"). Barley is an excellent source of soluble fiber and can help lower cholesterol. Eat it as a hot cereal, or use it in place of rice in a pilaf, risotto or casserole.

Beans and other legumes are a fabulous source of fiber and protein—not to mention phytochemicals such as protease inhibitors, which may prevent cancer. The options are endless: adzuki beans, Anasazi beans, black beans, chickpeas, great northern beans, lentils, split peas, lima beans, navy beans, pintos, red beans, and soybeans, for starters. If you've had trouble with gas after eating beans, try lentils and split peas, which are easiest to digest. Or look in your grocery store or drugstore's antacid section for a product called Beano, a natural enzyme that helps your body break down the complex sugars in some foods.

Buckwheat, like amaranth, isn't actually a cereal grain; it's more closely related to rhubarb. It contains a significant amount of the amino acid lysine. Use buckwheat grits as a breakfast cereal or rice-pudding-style dessert. Buckwheat groats (also called kasha) can be substituted for rice. Kasha can be added to soups, pilaf, or casseroles, and is excellent for stuffing meat, poultry, fish, or vegetables. Buckwheat flour makes a fantastic breakfast pancake.

Brown rice is just the whole-grain form of regular white rice. It takes longer to cook, and is a bit nuttier and chewier.

High-fiber breakfast cereals make a quick morning meal. Look for cereals that have at least five grams of fiber per serving.

Kamut, a form of wheat grown in ancient Egypt, has a rich, buttery flavor with a chewy texture. It's great as a hot or cold breakfast cereal, marinated in salads, or mixed with rice and beans.

Millet is a good source of B vitamins, copper and iron. The grain is delicate and bland, so it can be combined with most flavorings. Prepare it as a hot cereal, use it in a casserole, or incorporate it in meat loaf.

Oats and oatmeal are good sources of soluble and insoluble fiber. Oats offer impressive levels of iron and manganese and also supply good quantities of copper, folacin, vitamin E and zinc. A University of Maryland study showed that oat bran reduces cholesterol levels as efficiently as two widely prescribed cholesterol-lowering drugs. Eat oatmeal for breakfast. Use oats in muffins, cookies, and breads. Prepare a thick smoothie with oat bran, skim milk, and fruit. Toss plain toasted oats into a green salad, soup or dessert, or use them as breading for baked chicken or fish.

Popcorn can be a great snack. If you're using microwave popcorn, look for a low-fat variety.

Quinoa (pronounced KEEN-wah) isn't actually a grain but is related to the leafy vegetables spinach and chard. Higher in protein than other grains, quinoa is also a good source of iron and magnesium, potassium, and riboflavin. Delicate-tasting quinoa can be used in soups, salads, and casseroles, or in any dish that calls for rice. It's great in enchiladas.

Rye offers more protein, iron, and B vitamins than whole wheat. Rye has a robust flavor, so try cooking it with milder-tasting grains.

Spelt resembles wheat in appearance and nutritional composition, but spelt provides 30 percent more protein. Use it alone or with other grains, in pilafs, casseroles, stuffings, or hot breakfast cereals.

Whole-grain pastas taste great with your favorite sauces.

Whole-grain crackers pair nicely with low-fat cheese.

Whole-wheat breads should replace white breads whenever possible. Don't forget to try whole-wheat English muffins, pita bread, and (of course) tortillas.

Wild rice is actually a grass seed. It supplies about twice the protein of other rices.

Vegetables and Fruits

Research overwhelmingly shows that fruits and vegetables can boost your immune system, help you control your weight, and generally keep you healthy.

In 1948, scientists recruited 5,209 residents of Framingham, Massachusetts, to take medical tests and discuss their health in detail. Since then, the Framingham Heart Study has continued following those original participants, as well as their children and grandchildren, and has shaped how Americans think about preventing disease. Over and over again, Framingham researchers discovered the importance of eating fruits and vegetables. They have found, for instance, that a diet high in fruits and veggies, magnesium and potassium protects against osteoporosis. According to an article in the *Journal of the American Medical Association,* the Framingham residents with the highest fruit and vegetable consumption had a 31 percent lower risk of suffering an ischemic stroke. Researchers found that adding an additional fruit and vegetable each day lowered the risk of stroke by 6 percent.

Outside Framingham, scads of other studies demonstrate the benefits of a diet high in fruits and veggies. High consumption of vegetables, especially crucifers such as broccoli, has been associated with reduced risk of prostate cancer. Women who eat lots of fruits and vegetables have a lower risk of cardiovascular disease, especially myocardial infarctions. And researchers have found that eating alpha-carotene and lycopene—found, of course, in fruits and vegetables—significantly reduces the risk of lung cancer.

And so on.

You've probably already heard about these studies or others like them. But if you're like most Americans, you haven't yet changed your diet: In 2004, an AC Nielsen poll found that more than 85 percent of respondents said they weren't eating five servings of fruits and vegetables a day. (The latest USDA recommendations say you should eat nine.)

So no more excuses. Put fruits and veggies on your plate tonight.

A few favorites:

Vegetables

Artichokes cannot be eaten quickly. So sit back and relax and enjoy them, leaf by leaf.

Asparagus can be oven-roasted or stir-fried, but one of the best ways to cook it is to steam it upright, points in the air, in shallow water. That way, the delicate tips won't get soggy.

Broccoli is one of the healthiest foods you can eat. Along with vitamins and minerals, it also provides nitrogen compounds called indoles, which studies have shown to protect against some forms of cancer. Broccoli also contains beta carotene, vitamin C (16 percent more than an orange), calcium and cancer-fighting enzymes.

Brussels sprouts have the same cancer-inhibiting potential as their crucifer cousins cabbage, broccoli, and cauliflower. They are also a good vegetable source of protein, which accounts for a whopping 31 percent of their calories.

Cabbage of all kinds (red, green, savoy or bok choy) contains indoles and a good amount of fiber, along with vitamin C.

Carrots contain the antioxidant beta carotene, which has been shown to fight cancer and reduce the risk of stroke. One study by the USDA showed that participants who ate seven ounces of carrots a day for three weeks reduced their cholesterol by 11 percent. Try eating carrots with tomatoes, since lycopene enhances the body's ability to absorb beta carotene.

Cauliflower, yet another cruciferous vegetable, can reduce your risk of cancer. Try it mashed, like potatoes.

Cucumbers are full of fiber. Just one eight-inch cucumber provides 12 percent of the amount of fiber recommended for one's daily intake. A cucumber salad with onion and vinegar and sweetened with a touch of Splenda makes a refreshing treat.

Greens, such as romaine, radicchio, chicory, red leaf and green leaf, spinach, collards, and kale, are rich in chlorophyllin, an antioxidant that enhances the immune system. Greens make fabulous salads—just be sure to choose a light or reduced-fat dressing. Add fresh parsley to the salad for a boost in vitamin C and iron.

Eggplant is filling and provides a meaty texture, perfect for vegetarian lasagna or a vegetarian main dish.

Garlic contains a substance that interferes with the formation of blood clots and may help reduce cholesterol.

Mushrooms contain beta glucan, which stimulates the immune system.

Okra offers more than five grams of fiber per 3.5-ounce serving. It also contributes a good amount of vitamin C, folacin, B vitamins, magnesium, potassium and calcium. The liquid released by cooked okra can help thicken stews and soups.

Onions, with their allyl sulfides, may help lower blood pressure and cholesterol.

Peppers are excellent source of vitamin C and may be effective in protecting against cancer.

Pumpkin tastes great in soups, muffins and breads.

Sprouts have high water content and provide a delicious addition to salads and sandwiches. You can grow sprouts yourself at any time of year. The most familiar are mung, alfalfa and radish sprouts.

Summer squash, such as zucchini and crookneck, contains beta carotene—but only in the skin, so be sure to eat that part.

Sweet potatoes are filling, relatively low in calories (a five-inch sweet potato has only about 120), and are packed with beta carotene and vitamin C.

Tomatoes contain lycopene, an antioxidant more potent than vitamin C. Lycopene stimulates immune function and may slow degenerative diseases.

Winter squash, such as acorn, pumpkin, spaghetti and butternut, has darker flesh than the summer varieties and is more nutritious. Winter squash is a good source of complex carbohydrates and beta carotene.

Fruit

Apples are a great source of fiber—especially the soluble kind that helps lower cholesterol and blood sugars. Stored in a plastic bag in the crisper, apples can keep for up to six weeks.

Apricots contain impressive amounts of beta carotene and are good sources of vitamin C, iron and potassium. NASA officials made them an official part of the astronauts' diets on a number of space flights.

Avocados derive from 71 to 88 percent of their calories from fat, but it is mainly the healthy monounsaturated fat. Use in moderation: two tablespoons per serving.

Bananas have more potassium by weight than any fruit except the avocado.

Berries—including blackberries, blueberries, cranberries, raspberries, and strawberries—are low in calories (50 to 70 calories per one-cup serving), so they make a great snack or dessert replacement. The main nutrients found in berries are vitamin C, potassium and fiber.

Cherries are sources of phenolic compounds and other phytonutrients. Sour cherries are lower in calories and higher in vitamin C and beta carotene than sweet cherries.

Dates are loaded with potassium—and, for a fruit, with calories. Try eating three or four sweet-as-honey dates with just a dab of cottage cheese.

Grapes aren't high in nutritional content, but some varieties are good sources of vitamin C. Their natural sweetness and low calorie count make them a nice snack. Try frozen grapes for a sweet treat.

Grapefruit is filling, tasty and low in calories. Look for Texas red grapefruits such as Rio Red and Texas Star Ruby. They're especially sweet, and they contain significantly higher levels of lycopene, beta carotene and other phytonutrients than other grapefruit.

Kiwifruits are packed with nutrition. One large kiwi has more vitamin C than a cup of strawberries, and two small kiwifruits have as much dietary fiber as a cup of bran flakes. An enzyme present in kiwi makes the fruit a good meat tenderizer.

Lemons are rich in vitamin C, and lemon juice can help replace salt as a flavoring.

Mangoes contain bioflavonoids that aid the immune system.

Melons, with their high water content and low calorie count, are good sources of potassium, vitamin C, and beta carotene.

Nectarines can be substituted in any dish that calls for peaches or apricots. They bring eye-popping color and flavor to fruit salads, salsas, and chutneys.

Oranges have more to offer than just vitamin C. They also pack generous levels of folacin and provide calcium, potassium, thiamin, niacin, and magnesium. The white membrane under the skin holds more vitamin C than the flesh. It also contains most of the pectin, the soluble fiber thought to help reduce cholesterol.

Papaya is rich in vitamin C. Most people discard the seeds, but they are edible, with a spicy, pepperlike flavor. Use them as a garnish.

Peaches are the third most popular fruit grown in the United States, right behind apples and oranges. Peaches can be eaten out of hand as a snack, or cut up and added to salads, desserts, cereals, or cooked dishes. They contribute a good amount of vitamin C.

Pears shouldn't be peeled; most of their vitamin C lies in the skin. Try adding pear slices to a chicken sandwich or on a salad with blue cheese.

Pineapples, when fresh, contain an enzyme called bromelain, which breaks down protein. Fresh pineapple should not be mixed with yogurt or cottage cheese until immediately before serving, or the bromelain will begin to break down the protein in these foods. Take advantage of bromelain by including pineapple in marinades to tenderize meats and poultry. Use it to sweeten sweet potatoes, or throw it into a Chinese stir-fry. Pineapple with a scoop of lemon sorbet makes a delicious dessert.

Plums come in more than 140 varieties. Make a colorful plum salad, or add sliced plums to low-fat yogurt and wheat germ.

Dairy Products

Recent research shows that people who consume lots of calcium tend to gain less weight and have better body compositions. A twenty-four-week study published in *Obesity Research* showed that adults on a reduced-calorie diet who ate three to four servings of dairy foods each day lost significantly more weight than those who also cut calories but consumed few or no dairy foods. But as with every food, dairy calories must fit into your meal plan. Extra calories from any food, low-fat dairy or not, will be stored as fat.

These dairy products are great sources of calcium:

Light yogurt
Low-fat buttermilk
One percent or **skim milk**
Reduced-fat cheese such as Cabot, Alpine Lace, Laughing Cow, and Sargento
Reduced-fat cottage cheese
Reduced-fat ricotta cheese

Proteins

Protein is crucial to building and maintaining muscle. It also improves your immune system and protects against osteoporosis. Good sources of protein include:

Meat and Poultry

Beef. Choose a lean grade, such as "choice" or "select." And choose lean cuts such as sirloin and tenderloin.

Chicken, especially white meat, without the skin

Deli meat. Buy lean varieties, such as turkey, ham, roast beef, and chipped beef.

Eggs and **egg whites**

Fish and **shellfish** (see below)

Game such as buffalo, duck, pheasant, and ostrich

Lamb, as long as you stick to lean cuts such as the roast, chop, or leg

Pork. Look for fresh ham, Canadian bacon, tenderloin, and loin chop.

Meat substitutes

Soy (see below)

Turkey, especially the white meat

Veal. Look for lean chops.

Fish and Shellfish

As long as they're not fried, all fish and shellfish are great low-fat, protein-rich additions to your diet. But some fish and shellfish are especially good sources of omega-3 acids, which protect against heart disease and type 2 diabetes—and, studies indicate, may also help fight hypertension, autoimmune diseases, depression, and cancer. To get your omega-3s, look for:

Anchovies
Bass
Bluefish
Catfish
Herring
Mackerel
Mussels
Rockfish
Salmon
Sardines
Trout
Tuna

Soy

Soy products contain nutrients and phytonutrients that can powerfully benefit your health. To date, research on soy has shown that eating it improves your cardiovascular health, eases menopause, and helps prevent cancer and osteoporosis. Newer studies hint that it may help protect against diabetes and kidney disease, and that it aids in weight management. The Food and Drug Administration says that twenty-five grams of soy protein per day, as part of a diet low in saturated fat and cholesterol, may reduce the risk of heart disease.

Twenty-five grams sounds like a lot—and if your diet is like most Americans', you'll have to work a bit to consume that much every day. But as the number of soy-based products grows, it becomes easier to work soy into your diet. And more and more often, you can find soy products not only in health-food stores but on the shelves of regular grocery stores.

The following are common soy products and the amount of soy protein they provide:

Soy sausage link   6 grams
Eight-ounce glass plain soymilk   10 grams

Soy protein bar	14 grams
½ cup tempeh	16 grams
¼ cup soy nuts	12 grams

Some soy limitations need to be considered. Women being treated for breast cancer should not consume soy; research that shows that it may encourage cancer-cell proliferation. Also, those on thyroid medication should avoid consuming soy around the time that they take their medication, since the meds' efficacy can be affected. If you fall into either of those categories, discuss your diet with your physician.

The following are the most common sources of soy protein:

Tofu is made from cooked and pureed soybeans that are processed into a custardlike cake. Tofu has a neutral flavor and can be stir-fried, added to smoothies, or blended into cream cheese mixtures to use for dips. A four-ounce serving contains 13 grams of soy protein.

Soymilk is made by grinding hulled soybeans and mixing them with water. Soymilk can be drunk as a beverage or substituted in recipes for cow's milk. An eight-ounce glass contains ten grams of soy protein.

Textured soy protein is made from defatted soy flour, which is dehydrated. It can be used as a meat substitute or as a filler in dishes such as meat loaf.

Tempeh, made from whole, cooked soybeans formed into a chewy cake, can be used as a meat substitute.

Miso, fermented soybean paste, adds a pleasant, deep flavor to salad dressings and soups.

Soy protein isolate is extracted from the soybean in a process that retains about 90 percent of the protein. It's an economical source of protein and an easily digestible source of necessary amino acids. And besides, it's low in fat, calories and cholesterol.

Soy nuts can be eaten right out of your hand, like regular nuts.

Soy cheeses are just what they sound like: cheeses made from soymilk.

Herbs and Spices

Yes, you read that right. Just adding pizzazz to your plate can also add antioxidants to your diet.

Cinnamon has potent antioxidant properties that can help us fight against heart disease. Studies show that people consuming one-quarter to one teaspoon a day for forty days saw their total cholesterol levels drop by 13 to 26 percent; their LDL cholesterol (the bad kind) dropped 7 to 27 percent; and their triglycerides fell 23 to 30 percent. Cinnamon may help lower blood glucose levels, although this research is not yet conclusive.

Curry, a spice blend used widely in India, shows high antioxidant activity. Some research suggests that curry may help protect the brain from cancer, Alzheimer's disease, dementia, and aging. Curry goes well with wheat pasta, brown rice, chicken, turkey, fruit, beets, carrots, parsnips, winter squash, and sweet potatoes.

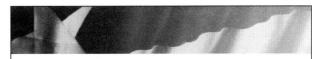

SOY: OH, BOY!

- Try soy-based beverages, muffins, sausages, yogurt or cream cheese for breakfast.
- Use soy deli meats, soy nut butter (similar to peanut butter), or soy cheese to make sandwiches.
- Top pizzas with soy cheese, soy pepperoni, soy sausages, or "crumbles" (similar to ground beef).
- Grill soy hot dogs, burgers, marinated tempeh and baked tofu.
- Cube and stir-fry tofu or tempeh and add to a salad.
- Use soymilk in place of regular milk. Pour soymilk on your cereal. Use it in your recipes. Or make smoothies.
- Order soy-based dishes such as spicy bean curd and miso soup at Asian restaurants.
- Eat roasted soy nuts or a soy protein bar for a snack.

Ginger has been used for medicinal purposes for centuries. Ginger is ideal for nausea related to pregnancy and chemotherapy, and is helpful in alleviating arthritic pain. A powerful antioxidant, ginger helps fight cancer. Try it with rice, chicken, duck, fruit, beets, salad dressing, carrots, winter squash, or sweet potatoes.

Oregano is powerful stuff. The U.S. Department of Agriculture found that just one tablespoon of fresh oregano possesses the antioxidant kick of an entire apple. Oregano tastes great in breads, deviled eggs, omelettes, chicken, beef, lamb, pork, veal, venison, cabbage, eggplant, and tomatoes.

Rosemary exhibits antioxidant, anti-inflammatory, and anti-carcinogenic activity. It's terrific with eggs, chicken, fish, beef, lamb, pork, veal, cauliflower, peas, and potatoes.

Turmeric is full of antioxidants and also works as an anti-inflammatory. India's elders say turmeric helps them remain sharp and clear-headed. It's commonly used in curries. But try it in deviled eggs, too.

Good Fats

Our bodies need fat. It stores energy, and is necessary for nutrient transport, growth, and as a component of many of cells. A totally fat-free diet may lead to continuous hunger and possible overeating—but, of course, most people don't have that problem.

As we all know, too much fat is bad—and it's easy to eat too much. Try to keep fat calories below 30 percent of your total calories. The majority of your fat intake should be the healthiest kind of fat, monounsaturated.

Sources of good fat include:

All-natural peanut butter
Avocados
Canola oil
Fish oil
Flaxseed oil
Nuts (almonds, cashews, peanuts, pecans)
Olive oil
Peanut oil
Sesame seeds
Trans-free margarines

Step up to the New Food Pyramid ... and a Healthier You!

The new food pyramid just released by the U.S. Department of Agriculture, "Steps to a Healthier You," is very much dancing in line with the *Texas Two-Step Diet.* Amy applauds its adoption and offers her personal adaptations:

Grains

6 ounces of breads, crackers and cereal, rice, or pasta—whole grains are best.

Vegetables

Include 2½ cups of vegetables every day—emphasize the dark-green and leafy vegetables. Orange is in! Try carrots, sweet potatoes, winter squash or pumpkin. Also try colorful sweet or hot peppers and fresh or dried beans, including lentils, pintos, kidneys, red beans, black-eyes and split green peas.

Fruits

We need 2 cups per day. Such a wide variety of fruits are available from national and worldwide sources ... apples, apricots, peaches, pears, plums, grapes, berries, bananas, pineapples, cherries and melons.

Milk and Dairy Products

3 cups per day. *Go low*—low-fat milk, yogurt and cottage cheese.

Meat and Beans

5½ ounces. Again, *go low* and choose low-fat, lean meats and poultry; find more fish; and include more high-protein beans, peas, seeds and nuts.

For more information, go to www.mypyramid.gov.

*In preparing for battle I have always found
that plans are useless,
but planning is indispensable.*

—Dwight D. Eisenhower

Chapter 9

Shopping for a Better Tomorrow

Action Point Seven:
Stock your pantry with the right stuff

Most of us throw boxes and bottles into our shopping cart without ever glancing at the nutrition labels. And that's a shame: Those labels give you a quick, easy way to compare the nutritional value of foods. So it's time you start peering at your groceries *before* you take them home.

Here's what to look for:

The **ingredient list** has a specific order: The first ingredient on the list is the one that's most predominant by weight, the second is the second most predominant, and so on. You want to be sure that harmful or empty ingredients—hydrogenated vegetable oil, corn syrup, and such—are low on the list, or better yet, not there at all.

Calories, yes, are those things that you count. Technically a calorie is a measure of energy—but, of course, if you consume more energy than you burn, that energy is stored as fat. And if you're trying to lose weight (no surprise here), you want to consume fewer calories than you burn.

The **serving size** is important, and it may surprise you. For instance, a box of cereal may list half a cup as the serving size, with a light-sounding 90 calories. But we know that we usually eat about one cup, so we're actually consuming 180 calories.

The **total fat** found in a serving includes all types of fat: monounsaturated, polyunsaturated, saturated, and trans fats. Saturated fat and trans fats are unhealthy, so you want to limit them as much as possible—and aim to eliminate them. When you're buying a product, make sure that the saturated fat is not the majority of the total fat. For instance, if the total fat is six grams, you'd want the saturated fat to be two grams or less.

Trans fats are perhaps the worst of all, but at present, it's hard to tell how much of them are hidden in a product's total fat. (Starting in 2006, FDA rules will require manufacturers' labels to list the amount of trans fats separately.) For now, check your ingredients list for the word "hydrogenated." And if you see it, especially near the top of the ingredient list, look for another product.

The 5-20 Rule

Labels don't list *every* nutrient—only the ones that relate to today's most pressing health issues. Some of those nutrients (fiber, vitamins A and C, calcium, and iron) are listed because Americans don't eat enough of them. And some (fat, saturated fat, cholesterol and sodium) are listed because we eat too much.

Most foods, though, have both good stuff and bad stuff. So how do you tell when a food is a nutritional good deal?

You turn to the 5–20 rule, which applies if you're consuming roughly 2,000 calories a day, *foods should provide 5 percent or less of the recommended daily allowance of nutrients, such as fat, that you want to limit. And they should provide 20 percent or more of the daily allowance of nutrients you need.*

The Magic Number 30

In general, you want fat to make up less than 30 percent of your daily intake of calories. To figure out quickly whether a product fits a healthy diet, use the Magic Number 30 Fat Test: Take the number of fat grams and multiply it by 30 (the magic number). Then check whether the answer is the same or lower than the number of calories per serving. If it is, the product is low in fat—and thus eligible to be dropped in your cart.

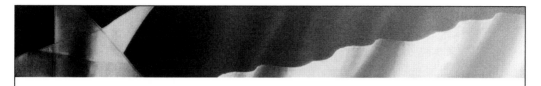

FOOD FOR THOUGHT

- Look for small pieces of fruit. They're often sweeter than larger pieces of the same fruit.
- Freeze grapes or sliced bananas for a healthy sweet treat.
- Use Benecol Light, Take Control Light or Smart Balance as a healthy alternative to butter or margarine. These cholesterol-lowering spreads contain either plant stanol esters or plant sterol esters— both of which have been proven to help lower cholesterol. Benecol Light is heat-stable and can be used in cooking.
- If you're worried about feeling hungry, plan to incorporate filling but light water-rich foods into your meal. Soup with dinner works great!
- Plan to leave a bowl of cut-up fruit in a highly visible spot in the refrigerator. If it's convenient, tempting, and easily accessible, you'll be more likely to use it as a snack.
- Store cleaned, cut-up vegetables in a clear container in the refrigerator as a reminder to use them.
- Make yogurt cheese to use as a creamy low-fat base for dips, cracker spreads, salad dressings, and soups. Line a strainer with cheesecloth or a coffee filter, place the strainer over a bowl, add gelatin-free yogurt, and cover. As liquid drips out of the yogurt, the yogurt takes on a firmer, cheesier texture. Strain for two to twenty-four hours, depending on the firmness you desire.

For example, let's say that a serving of cereal contains 3 grams of fat and 90 calories per serving. You multiply the number of fat grams (3) by the magic number (30). The answer, 90, is the same as the number of calories per serving. So your cereal is okay.

But let's say that another cereal contains 6 grams of total fat and 90 calories. You would calculate 6 × 30, and find that the answer, 180, is far greater than 90, and therefore not a great choice to bring home.

Like most rules, the Magic Number 30 has exceptions. There will be times when a food product will fail the fat test, but because the majority or all of the fat comes from the healthiest type of fat available (monounsaturated), it is acceptable to eat in moderation.

For example, let's look at peanut butter. Peter Pan, Jif, and Skippy have similar labels: For a serving size of 2 tablespoons, they have 180 calories and 16 total grams of fat. And 16 × 30=480, which is significantly greater than 180. So the major brands fail the first round of the fat test.

Now if you go look at the ingredient list you will also find the word "hydrogenated," which means that the peanut butter has trans fat. And that word "hydrogenated" appears high on the ingredient list, usually in the second spot. So not only do these peanut butters flunk the Magic Number 30 test, but they also contain unhealthy trans fats. So Peter Pan, Jif, and Skippy should not find their way to your pantry shelf.

Now, let's look at all-natural peanut butters such as I.M. Healthy, Smuckers All Natural or even soy-nut butter or almond butter. The nutrition labels will be the same or very similar to the big commercial brands: Serving size 2 tablespoons, calories 180, total fat 16 grams. So even these health-store versions flunk the first round of the fat test.

But this time, when you look at the ingredient lists, you won't find the word "hydrogenated." Because peanuts and almonds are rich sources of monounsaturated fats (a good kind of fat), and nothing else has been added to this product, we can consume it in moderation.

"In moderation" is the tricky part. Too much of even a good thing is no longer a good thing.

Remember that your food's effect on your body is cumulative, and that what you eat today will have repercussions for years to come. It's estimated that by the time a person reaches age sixty-five, he will have consumed fifty tons of food and drink—and it matters whether that tonnage was healthy food and drink or junk.

As Dr. Ken Cooper says, "It's easier to maintain our health than to regain it."

Checking for Quality Carbs

Not all carbohydrates are created equal. But how do you tell the good ones from the junk? With this rule of thumb: *The more fiber, the better the carb.*

For this rule you'll check the label for "total carbohydrates" and "dietary fiber." With starchy foods, you want to ensure that the carbohydrate content includes at least a little fiber.

- A serving of bread, crackers, rice or pasta should contain *at least* two grams of fiber.
- A serving of breakfast cereal should contain *at least* five grams of fiber.

Stocking Your Kitchen

Okay, okay—life is short, and you can't read every label in the store on every shopping trip. So first concentrate on the stuff that you already buy. Before your next grocery-store trip, you might want to assess some of the foods you have in your home. Go through the refrigerator and pantry and decide which products are fine, and which shouldn't be restocked.

Now make your grocery list, using your food lists from chapter 8—and, if you like, with the list below of products that meet the rules of thumb.

Pantry

Apple cider vinegar
Balsamic vinegar
Beans, canned or dried
Breakfast cereals with more than five grams of fiber per serving
Canola oil
Chicken, canned in water
Chicken broth
Herbs and spices (Mrs. Dash seasoning, Molly McButter sprinkles)
Nonfat cooking spray such as Pam
Nuts (almonds are fantastic)
Oat bran hot cereal
Oatmeal
Olive oil
Popcorn (low-fat, if buying the microwave kind)
Rice (brown or wild)
Salsa
Soups (bean and veggie; check for low-sodium varieties if you have high blood pressure)
Soy nuts
Soy or whey protein powders (for smoothies)

Spaghetti sauce
Textured vegetable protein
Tofu
Tomatoes (canned, paste or puree)
Tuna, packed in water
Whole-grain bread products (bread, muffins, pitas, tortillas)
Whole-wheat pastas (including couscous)
Wholesome flours (buckwheat, oat, rye, whole-wheat pastry flour, graham, soy)
Wholesome grains (amaranth, barley, buckwheat, oats, quinoa)

Refrigerator

Applesauce (unsweetened)
Broccoli sprouts
Cheese (reduced-fat)
Cottage cheese (low-fat)
Deli meat (the lean kind)
Fruits (whatever's in season)
Garlic
Ground flaxseed
I Can't Believe It's Not Butter spray
Lemon juice
Lettuce (the dark, leafy kind)
Mayonnaise (reduced-fat)
Meat alternatives (Gardenburgers, soy sausage, soy ground beef, soy hot dogs)
Milk (low-fat or skim)
Mustard
Soymilk
Vegetables (whatever's in season)
Yogurt (light)

Freezer

Buffalo
Chicken breast

Edamame
Fish
Fruit (frozen in bags)
Ground meat (lean)
Meat substitutes
Tofu
Veggies (frozen in bags)

Recommended Brands

We're offering this list as a convenient shortcut, so you don't have to read every label in the store. But if a food meets the rules of thumb, don't worry if the brand isn't on this list. We couldn't possibly include everything.

Baking Products

Arrowhead Mills flours and mixes
Bob's Red Mill flours
Hodgson Mill flours and mixes

Breads

Food for Life Ezekiel Bread
Nature's Own Wheat N Fiber
Natural Ovens (many varieties)
Oroweat Carb Control
Vitamuffins (vitalicious.com)

Butter Substitutes

Benecol Light (contains plant sterols that help lower cholesterol)
Smart Balance spray
Molly McButter
Smart Balance (and other butter sprays that contain no trans fats)
Take Control Light (contains plant sterols that help lower cholesterol)

Cereals

Barbara's Bakery Grain Shop
Barbara's Bakery Organic Soy Essence
Barbara's Bakery Puffins—Cinnamon
General Mills Fiber One
General Mills Total Raisin Bran
Health Valley Fiber 7 Flakes
Kashi Good Friends
Kashi Heart to Heart
Kashi GoLean!
Kellogg's All-Bran
Kellogg's Raisin Bran
Post Cinna-Cluster Raisin Bran
Post Bran Flakes
Uncle Sam

Cheese

Alpine Lace
Athenos reduced-fat feta
Cabot 50% or 75% light
Frigo light cheese sticks
Jarlsberg light
Kraft reduced-fat shredded cheddar and mozzarella
Laughing Cow Light part-skim ricotta
Sargento light string cheese

Chips

Guiltless Gourmet
Lays Baked Chips
Skinny

Crackers

Ak-Mak
Finn Crisp
Hain Honey/Cinnamon Grahams
Health Valley graham crackers
Kashi TLC
Ryvita
Wasa

Frozen Meals

Frozen meals vary greatly, so even with these usually reliable brands, be sure to perform a fat test and check for fiber. And if you have high blood pressure, watch the sodium content.

Create a Meal, Green Giant, stir-fry varieties
Healthy Choice
Lean Cuisine
Stouffer's Lean Cuisine
Van de Kamp's Crisp & Healthy baked breaded fish fillets
Weight Watchers
Wolfgang Puck's grilled vegetable cheese-less pizza

Meat Alternatives

Boca Burger Chik'n Patties, Italian sausage, breakfast links, original ground burger
Gardenburgers
Lightlife Smart Ground, Gimme Lean Sausage Style
Loma Linda
Mori-Nu Tofu
Morningstar Farms
Smart Dogs
Tofu Pups
White Wave tempeh
White Wave tofu

Seasonings and Dips

Athenos hummus
Mrs. Dash
Pam olive-oil cooking spray

Soy Snacks

Genisoy Soy Crisps
Genisoy Soy Nuts
Skinny Soy Chips

Tortillas

La Tortilla Factory

Yogurts

Blue Bunny carb-control yogurt
Blue Bunny lite yogurt
Dannon Light 'n Fit Smoothies and yogurts
Stonyfield Farm yogurt and smoothies (Bonus: They contain inulin, a natural fiber that helps promote digestive health and boosts calcium absorption.)
Yoplait Ultra

Remember: Above all else, your shopping cart *must* be full of fruits and vegetables. For those you don't need brand-name recommendations, just plenty of vibrant colors!

Alternative to Action Point Seven

If you're not ready to change the way you shop, at least try *some* of the new foods suggested. Experiment! Have fun!

Attack Your Snacks!

Keep healthy snacks available: nonfat yogurt, washed, fresh fruits and veggies and unsalted nuts in a place where they're easily seen and picked up. These snacks will satisfy the need for something crunchy, creamy or sweet as well as a protein boost, depending on your specific craving.

If you have to have chips, buy the baked versions … but the better choice is to bake your own.

Baked Potato Chips

Slice baking potatoes into rounds, getting them as thin as you can. (Sprinkle with parmesan if you like.) Bake at 350° for 30–45 minutes, watching so they don't burn. (Note: Try substituting carrots or sweet potatoes for baking potatoes.)

Baked Tortilla Chips

Cut corn tortillas into strips, triangles or use cookie cutters with your kids to make fun shapes. Bake for 7–8 minutes in a 300° oven. Sprinkle with a little salt or salt substitute, if desired.

Boursin Cheese Dip

8 oz. package of nonfat cream cheese
½ cup nonfat yogurt or nonfat cottage cheese
1 T. fresh parsley and/or cilantro, chives or oregano
1 T. Dijon mustard
1 tsp. chopped garlic
1 T. grated Parmesan
Salt to taste

Serve with baked chips, whole-wheat crackers or melba toast.

I love Texas because Texas is future-oriented, because Texans think anything is possible. Texans think big.

—Phil Gramm

Chapter 10

Supplements?

I t's not surprising that Texans gravitate toward nutritional supplements—vitamins, minerals, herbs, amino acids, hormones, whatever you've got. We're big-state, big-thinking people who love bigness in a big way. Supplements promise us speed and bold strokes. If 100 percent of your recommended daily allowance is good, we reason, isn't 200 percent twice as good? Heck, why not go for 1000 percent? Why settle for the puny amounts of good stuff contained naturally in food?

Watch out, because that line of thinking leads to a diet of nothing but pills—and to bad health. Scientists are still unraveling the complicated reactions between the chemicals that give fruits and vegetables their immune-boosting punch. For the time being, at least, the *only* way to guarantee your daily dose of free-radical busters is to eat a balanced, varied diet.

But supplements *do* have their place. Start by thinking of a supplement as just that: a supplement. It's not a food. It's not a drug. It's not supposed to replace nutrients you ought to get from food. And it won't fix problems brought on by years of poor dietary choices.

Think of a dietary supplement as an insurance policy. Insurance is useful to cover gaps, but you first need to protect yourself the best you can. Eating a healthy real-food diet is like stopping at red lights or looking both ways before you cross the street. Sure, you *could* rely on your insurance. But wouldn't you rather stay out of the hospital?

Of course, accidents and bad-nutrition days *do* happen. And when they do, there's something to be said for a good insurance policy—or its nutritional equivalent, a daily multivitamin.

Shopping for a Multivitamin

You want to look for a multivitamin that provides 100 percent of your daily requirement of the nutrients listed.

Be careful about overdoing things: Sometimes exceeding 100 percent of the guidelines can be dangerous. Too much retinol from vitamin A can be toxic to your liver. Beta carotene, which the body converts to vitamin A, does not carry the same risk. If you are male or a postmenopausal woman, you more than likely do not need 100 percent of the recommended daily allowance of iron—and three times the recommended daily allowance could cause organ damage. Excessive vitamin B6 can cause nerve damage (though it is, thankfully, reversible). And so on. The bottom line is this: Meeting the recommended daily allowance is fine, but before you take a megadose, be sure you know what you're doing.

And that, of course, is just for the vitamins listed on the FDA labels. Health-food shelves are crowded with other supplements backed with far less research. Should you take glucosamine? Garlic pills? DHEA? Creatine? Coenzyme Q10? Some of the things on the shelves might work, some of these might work for certain people under certain conditions, and some are almost certainly snake oil—and expensive, potentially harmful snake oil at that.

So watch out. Surveys report that more than 40 percent of Americans take some form of dietary supplement, and in Amy's practice, about half of new clients say they're taking something. Often new clients rattle off a laundry list of supplements, but can't explain *why* they're taking those pills. Most say that a friend or the media convinced them that they should take the supplement, but they can't remember why—or maybe they never knew in the first place.

So do your research. And be careful: There's a lot of bad information out there, be it word of mouth, sloppy media reports, or Internet sites. Don't depend on the results of just a single study, and make especially sure that you're not relying only on the manufacturer's claims.

And *don't* trust a bottle's label. Many supplements are labeled inaccurately. Although the Food and Drug Administration requires food and drugs to be tested for safety, it does *not* require testing for supplements. Too often, what's stated on the label may not match what's actually in the bottle.

There is, however, an organization you can trust. U.S. Pharmacopeia (USP) is an independent organization that administers a dietary supplement verification program. Manufacturers who comply are able to display the letters "USP" on their products. The USP code means that the product meets the following guidelines:

1. It contains the ingredients listed on the label.
2. It contains the declared amount of ingredients listed.
3. It will dissolve effectively to release nutrients to the body.
4. It has been screened for harmful contaminants.
5. It was manufactured under safe and sanitary conditions.

Note that all multivitamins are not created equal. Some may contain unnecessary herbs and ineffective amounts of phytonutrients, which only waste your money.

The following are some basic guidelines to follow when selecting a multivitamin.

Vitamin A

Needed for healthy eyes and skin.
- **100% of the FDA-recommended daily requirement:** 5,000 IU
- Try to get at least 20% as beta carotene.
- **Safe upper limit:** 10,000 IU

Vitamin C

Helps keep the immune system strong.
- **100% daily requirement:** 60 mg
- Smokers need about 200 percent of the recommended daily allowance, or 120 mg. (Better yet, stop smoking.)
- If you have recurring kidney stones, avoid doses over 100 mg.
- **Safe upper limit:** 2,000 mg. Diarrhea and cramping may occur with higher doses.

Vitamin D

Makes it possible for you to absorb calcium from your food.
- **100% daily requirement:** 400 IU
- If you're over age 70, take an extra 200 IU (600 IU total) in a separate supplement.
- **Safe upper limit:** 2,000 IU

Vitamin E

Squelches free radicals that foster heart disease. Natural vitamin E is better than synthetic.
- **100% daily requirement:** 30 IU
- Consider taking 100 to 400 IU of vitamin E. Some multivitamins contain extra E, or you may need a separate supplement.
- If you are taking anticoagulant medications, make sure your doctor monitors your vitamin E intake.
- **Safe upper limit:** 1,500 IU natural; 1,100 IU synthetic

Vitamin K

Essential for your blood to clot.
- **100% daily requirement:** 80 mcg
- **Safe upper limit:** 30,000 mcg

Thiamin (B1)

Helps turn carbohydrates into energy.
- **100% daily requirement:** 1.5 mg
- **Safe upper limit:** 50 mg

Riboflavin (B2)

Needed for energy production in all your cells.
- **100% daily requirement:** 1.7 mg
- **Safe upper limit:** 200 mg

Niacin (B3)

Helps your body use sugar and fats.
- **100% daily requirement:** 20 mg
- **Safe upper limit:** 35 mg (unless by prescription)

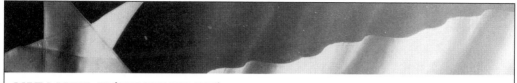

VITAMIN K(NOWLEDGE)

- Multivitamins don't have to be expensive. Read the label on store brands. Many are fine—and much cheaper than name brands.
- Watch out for unnecessary herbs. Many don't really add much nutritional value but do add a lot to the price.
- You may have heard that white marks on your nails indicate a vitamin deficiency. It's not true. They're caused by injury to the nail.
- Planning for surgery. Some supplements can cause complications such as bleeding, heart instability, low blood sugar, and blood-pressure changes. The American Society of Anesthesiologists recommends you avoid all supplements for two or three weeks before your hospital date.
- Have you heard that antacids can serve as calcium supplement? It's true—but avoid antacids with aluminum hydroxides, which hinder calcium absorption.

Pyridoxine (B6)

Used in making antibodies that fight infection.
- **100% daily requirement:** 2 mg
- **Safe upper limit:** 100 mg

Folic acid

Critical for making perfect DNA copies in new cells.
- **100% daily requirement:** 400 mcg
- **Safe upper limit:** 1,000 mcg

Vitamin B12

Keeps nerves healthy.
- **100% daily requirement:** 6 mcg
- **Safe upper limit:** 3,000 mcg

Iron

Helps the red blood cells carry oxygen.
- **100% daily requirement:** 18 mg
  Postmenopausal women and all men: 0 to 8 mg
- **Safe upper limit:** 45 mg

Iodine

Part of a thyroid hormone that regulates the rate at which you burn energy.
- **100% daily requirement:** 150 mcg
- **Safe upper limit:** 1,100 mcg

Zinc

Important for a strong immune system and for healing wounds.
- **100% daily requirement:** 15 mg
- **Safe upper limit:** 40 mg

Selenium

Helps knock out free radicals that may cause cancer.
- **100% daily requirement:** 70 mcg
- **Safe upper limit:** 400 mcg

Copper

Needed for healthy blood vessels and immune system.

- **100% daily requirement:** 2 mg (not as copper oxide or cupric oxide)
- **Safe upper limit:** 10 mg

Chromium

Works with insulin to help your body use blood sugar.
- **100% daily requirement:** 120 mcg
- **Safe upper limit:** 1,000 mcg

Shopping for Other Supplements

Some crucial nutrients usually aren't available in multivitamins—often because including 100 percent of the FDA-recommended daily requirement would make the pills too huge to swallow. But you might still want to consider taking these as separate supplements.

Calcium

Helps make strong bones, fights high blood pressure.
- For best absorption, don't take more than 500 mg of calcium at a time.
- If you're under 50, consider taking 500 mg calcium as a separate supplement.
- If you're over 50, consider taking 700 mg, in at least two separate doses.
- **Safe upper limit:** 2,500 mg

Magnesium

For strong bones, healthy nerves and muscles.
- **What to look for:** About 100 mg
- **Safe upper limit:** 350 mg

Potassium

Helps fight high blood pressure.
- **What to look for:** About 40 mg
- **Safe upper limit:** 99 mg (unless by prescription)

Fort Worth has more doughnut shops per capita than any other city in our survey— about four times the national average.

— *"America's Fattest Cities 2005," Men's Health Magazine*

Chapter 11

What *Not* to Eat

Action Point Eight:
Get rid of the bad, and don't overdo the good stuff

Now that good food is waiting in your kitchen, it's time to stop eating the bad stuff: the junk food, the empty calories, the items high in fat and sugar and low in nutrients and fiber. We'll call those the Not Today Foods—both because they're downright no good, and because you want to avoid them today.

The trick to getting Not Today Foods out of your life? Don't try to stop everything at once. Remember: You're not on a crash diet. You're changing your life.

For week one, list three Not Today Foods that you eat frequently. You know what we're talking about. Write them down—we'll call this your Not Today List—and promise yourself not to allow those health-wrecking substances into your mouth under any circumstances for the next 24 hours. It's not that hard, is it, just avoiding three foods? You have that kind of willpower, don't you? (When you don't, it's time to call your Two-Step Partner.)

For week two, add two more foods to your Not Today List, bringing your total to five. Last week you managed three; this time you're adding only two. You can do this. Believe in yourself, and you'll be able to follow through.

For week three, add two more Not Today Foods to your list, again with the same conditions. You now have seven items on your list.

For week four, add two more nutrition-busters to this list, for a total of nine.

For week five, add one last Not Today Food. You have finished your top ten, and you can probably already tell how much your body thanks you.

Good Riddance

Here's what a real-life Not Today List might look like.
Week One
1. French fries
2. Bacon
3. Doughnuts and sweet rolls

Week Two
4. Cakes and pies
5. White bread

Week Three
6. Butter or margarine
7. Soft drinks

Week Four
8. Sugary cereals
9. High-fat beef

Week Five
10. Jif, Peter Pan and Skippy peanut butter

Enough, But Not Too Much

Once you're eating good foods, it's time to think about quantity as well as quality. Texans, even more than most Americans, are eating super-size portions—huge amounts of food relative to what people ate even a decade ago. And our waistlines have adjusted.

Paul Rozin, a psychology researcher at the University of Pennsylvania, was interested in the "French paradox": Although the French diet oozes fatty foods such as croissants, foie gras and Brie, only 7 percent of the French are obese.

Rozin suspected that part of the difference between American and French waistlines lay in serving sizes. He compared meal sizes in Philadelphia restaurants, cookbooks, and super-markets to their counterparts in Paris. His finding: The French eat much smaller servings.

In pizzerias, ice cream parlors, bistros and ethnic restaurants, portions were 25 percent larger in Philly than in Paris.

In cookbooks, American meat-based recipes yielded servings 53 percent larger than their French counterparts; and veggie-based recipes made servings that were 25 percent smaller.

In the supermarket, the U.S. sizes were overall 37 percent larger than the French versions of the same food. American oranges were 42 percent larger; sodas, 52 percent; hot dogs, 63 percent; and yogurt, 82 percent.

Rozin also compared the time it takes to complete meals at an American McDonald's and at a McDonald's in Paris. He found that though Americans were eating significantly more food,

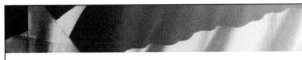

TAKING CONTROL

Eating Out

- Instead of an entrée, order a healthy appetizer.
- Split an entrée with a friend. Most restaurant meals are more than enough for two.
- Ask your server to bring a doggie bag when delivering your meal. When the meal arrives, immediately put half the food in the bag to take home.
- Ask your server to not bring chips or bread prior to the meal.
- Ask for a half portion.
- Make good substitutions, such as steamed veggies for anything fried, or a sweet potato instead of a baked potato.

they consumed their meals much faster: in 14.4 minutes in Philadelphia, versus 22 minutes in Paris.

So this is what the French have to teach us: Eat more slowly. Eat less. Enjoy it more.

Portions are especially a problem in restaurants, which take pride in serving us more for our money. We love our Tex-Mex baskets of tortilla chips, and the free bread that appears at steak houses (as if a towering hunk of beef and a baked potato the size of a football weren't enough). It's estimated that Americans eat 40 percent of their meals away from home, so those aren't just occasional indiscretions.

What to do? Take control of your portions, wherever you're eating.

> What's the difference between "portion" and a "serving"? A portion is how much of something you actually eat in one sitting. A serving is a standard size dictated by the United States Department of Agriculture and by the Food and Drug Administration for the nutrition labels on food packages.
>
> For instance, the food pyramid defines a serving of pasta as ⅓ cup. You read that right: a measly ⅓ cup. But who eats only ⅓ cup of pasta? Let's say you eat a whole cup: That's three servings, but one portion.

Extra food means extra calories, of course. And over time, cutting out just a few calories a day can have a huge effect on your waistline. The chart below shows how many pounds you'd gain each year if you consumed one more item each day in addition to meeting your caloric needs.

Food Item	Additional Calories	Weight Gain in One Year
Energy bar	250	26 pounds
Grande skim latte	160	17 pounds
12-ounce soda	140	15 pounds
½ cup light ice cream	120	12.5 pounds
20 pretzels	110	11.5 pounds
½ cup Raisin Bran	95	10 pounds
3.5 oz. white wine	70	7 pounds
3 Triscuits	60	6 pounds
1 T. mayo	45	5 pounds

Alternative to Action Point Eight

Instead of getting rid of ten kinds of Not Today Food, select a smaller number. You'll probably find that it's not as big a sacrifice as you imagine—and you can always cut out more in the future.

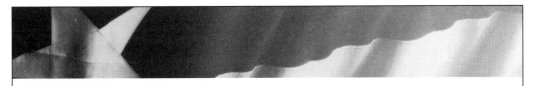

TAKING CONTROL

At Home

- Use smaller plates and bowls. It's natural to fill them up, and the same amount of food looks larger when it's on a small plate.
- Put food on your plates while you're in the kitchen, then put the food away. Putting food on the table makes it easy and tempting to have seconds even when you're no longer hungry.
- Portion out leftovers into individual serving-size containers to use for lunches or a later meal.
- Never eat out of a bag or carton.
- Always sit down while you eat.
- Never eat in front of the television. While your mind is on the TV, it's easy to devour an entire bag of Doritos.
- Designate eating places—for instance, the dining room table, the breakfast bar in your kitchen, or the picnic table in your backyard—and do not allow yourself to eat anywhere else when you're home.
- If you have trouble knowing when to stop, buy individualized servings, such as ice cream sandwiches instead of cartons of ice cream.
- When you get home from the grocery store, immediately divide large bags of snacks—pretzels, chips, etc.—into small individual-serving-size Ziploc baggies.
- Never snack while standing in front of an open refrigerator.

Obesity is a weighty issue in Texas:
More than 1 out of 4 adults is clinically
obese, according to the CDC. More than 6
out of 10 are at risk for health problems
because of their weight, and almost
3 out of 10 haven't been physically active
at all for the past 30 days.

—"America's Fattest Cities 2005,"
Men's Health Magazine

Chapter 12

Still *More* Reasons to Eat Right

Amy often finds herself saying to clients, "If only you could see the research that comes across my desk every day stating the power of a wholesome diet consisting of fruits, vegetables, low-fat dairy, and whole grains in the diet, you would be astonished." And maybe you'd be motivated. With that in mind, let's look at just some of that research.

- For men who already have symptoms of heart disease, two carrots every other day provide enough beta carotene to reduce stroke risk by half.
- One cup of uncooked spinach contains vitamins A and C, plus folic acid and magnesium. Eating spinach can help prevent cancer from developing, reduce one's risk for heart disease, and block many of the free radicals that can cause osteoporosis. Spinach is also rich in the antioxidants beta carotene and lutein. Although the actual amounts look fairly small, spinach contains far more of these two combined than any other fruit or vegetable.
- Strawberries contain ellagic acid, which has anti-cancer properties.
- Mangoes contain bioflavonoids that aid the immune system.
- Citrus fruits have vitamin C, which helps fight cancer.
- Papaya, pineapple and kiwi have high amounts of enzymes that help combat autoimmune disease, allergies, and cancer.
- Garlic may help lower blood pressure and cholesterol.

- Onion and shallots offer sulfur-containing compounds that help prevent cancer.
- Researchers at the University of Utah have found that high intakes of fruits, vegetables, and whole grains reduce the risk of rectal cancer by roughly 30 percent each, while high intake of refined grains increases risk of rectal cancer by 42 percent.
- Though nuts are high in total fat, they mostly contain monounsaturated and polyunsaturated fats—the good kinds. Many studies show that people who consume nuts regularly may be reducing their risk of heart disease. Scientific evidence suggests (but does not prove) that eating approximately ⅓ cup of nuts per day as part of a diet low in saturated fat and cholesterol may reduce the risk of heart disease.
- Research also has shown that many who consume nuts are not gaining weight, perhaps because nuts help you feel full longer.
- Regular and varied consumption of fruits and vegetables reduces the risk of many kinds of cancer. They don't cure cancer, but they do appear to prevent it, and can also slow the early stages of tumor development.
- Some compounds in fruits and veggies, called plant hormones, resemble human hormones. A diet with plenty of fruits and vegetables may help compensate for the loss of estrogen during menopause and help prevent osteoporosis.
- By eating at least five servings of fruits and vegetables every day, it's estimated that we can prevent at least 20 percent of all cancers.
- Vitamin K is needed for osteocalcin, a protein required for good bone strength. You can get vitamin K by eating dark leafy greens, broccoli, asparagus, and cauliflower.
- The phytonutrient quercetin may help prevent oxidation of LDLs (bad cholesterol) and help prevent cancer and cataracts. Quercetin is found in red onions, the skin of apples, tea, red wine, broccoli, kale, berries, oranges, and tomatoes.
- Researchers say the best edible insurance for reducing the risk of the nation's three leading causes of death is to consume a diet that is rich in fruits and vegetables and high in fiber.
- Recent research shows that a diet low in zinc can impair our immune function. Get your zinc by eating beans, whole grains, wheat germ, lean meats and seafood.
- Studies confirm that eating fish protects against heart attacks. Aim for at least two servings of fatty fish (tuna, salmon, and the like) each week.

- Approximately 75 percent of soy's benefits are attributed to isoflavones, which fight cancer, strengthen our bones, and decrease the risk of heart attack. Aim for at least one or two servings of soy each day.
- Research shows that a cup of red beans has as many flavonoids as a glass of red wine. The soluble fiber in beans helps lower cholesterol levels.
- Researchers at Case Western Reserve University School of Medicine are studying people genetically at risk for Alzheimer's disease because they carry one or two copies of the ApoE gene (often called the Alzheimer's gene). About one in four people has this gene, which is associated with late-onset Alzheimer's disease, diagnosed at age 70 or older. About half the people who carry the gene

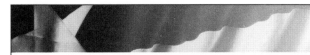

RELIABLE SOURCES (EVEN ON THE WEB)

Good sources of health news include:
- *The Washington Post's* health column, The Lean Plate Club. Look for it weekly at www.washingtonpost.com, or sign up to receive it via e-mail.
- www.nutrition.gov
- www.everydaychoices.org
- www.vitality.com
- www.cspinet.org
- www.webmd.com
- www.runnersworld.com
- www.mayoclinic.com
- www.vrg.org
- www.mypyramid.gov

actually develop the disease. Researchers found that people who have the gene and eat a high-fat diet during their forties are seven times more likely to develop the disease than those who do not carry the gene. When these genetically predisposed people ate a low-fat diet, their risk of developing the disease dropped to four and a half times that of those without the gene.
- The Mediterranean diet favored for centuries in places such as Italy and Greece is full of good stuff: fruits, vegetables, grains, legumes, nuts, cereals, and olive oil. The diet is moderate in fish intake and has less meat and dairy than the typical

American diet. Red wine is frequently drunk at dinner. It's not surprising that study after study has demonstrated its health benefits.

For four years, researchers from Greece followed some 22,000 adults aged twenty to eighty-six, tracking how closely they adhered to the typical Mediterranean diet. They found that those who stuck to the diet cut their risk of heart disease by 33 percent and cancer by 24 percent, compared to volunteers who ate other foods. The overall death rate dropped by 25 percent.

In June 2003, the *New England Journal of Medicine* published one of the largest studies ever done on the Mediterranean diet; it found that the diet's famous health contributions are attributable not only to the olive oil but to the diet as a whole. Still, give the olive oil its due: Penn State researchers found that three weeks of eating diets high in monounsaturated fat and low in saturated fat made subjects' LDL cholesterol (the bad kind) drop by 14 percent and triglycerides drop by 13 percent.

- The New American Plate, designed by the American Institute for Cancer, shows what your meal plate should look like. A variety of vegetables, fruits, whole grains and beans cover two-thirds of the plate. The remaining third of the plate contains meat or low-fat dairy.

- Two major studies have shown the effectiveness of DASH, the National Heart, Lung and Blood Institute's Dietary Approach to Stop Hypertension, a diet high in fruits, vegetables, and dairy foods, but low in saturated fat and total fat. DASH was found to lower blood pressure as well as diuretic drugs.

  For more information, go to www.nhlbi.nih.gov/health/public/heart/hbp/dash/.

- Researchers from the University of Toronto found that the Portfolio Diet, funded by the Almond Board of California, was as effective at lowering cholesterol levels as taking a strong dose of statin drugs. In three separate studies, people with high LDLs (bad cholesterol) ate a combination of vegetarian foods, including 1 ounce of almonds, 20 grams of viscous fiber foods, 2 grams of plant sterols and 50 grams of soy each day. In just four weeks, LDL cholesterol levels decreased by up to 35 percent, and LDL-to-HDL cholesterol ratios decreased by 30 percent—results similar to those of first-line cholesterol-lowering drugs.

  For more information, go to www.portfoliodiet.com.

Pot Roast

Yes, you can have your favorite pot roast and eat it, too! We have skimmed the fat off and made a gravy—yes, gravy—with the de-fatted pan juices thickened with vegetables to serve along side the sliced pot roast. The key is to cook the roast completely 2–24 hours before serving.

    1 3–4 pound boneless lean pork or beef roast (blade or cross rib, arm or round),
        fat trimmed
Kosher salt and freshly ground black pepper
2–3 T. vegetable oil
3 carrots, coarsely chopped
3 celery ribs, coarsely chopped
1 small yellow onion, peeled and coarsely chopped
1 large garlic clove, peeled and coarsely chopped
2 cups water, broth, red or white wine or some combination
½ cup Italian parsley leaves

Preheat the oven to 325°. Season meat very well with salt and pepper, rubbing seasoning into the meat evenly. Let seasoned meat sit for 30 minutes.

Heat oil in large roasting pan over medium-high heat. Dry the roast well with paper towels. Add the meat to the pan and brown on all sides, being careful not to scorch it.

About halfway through the browning process, add the carrot, celery, onion and coarsely chopped garlic and let the vegetables brown a little.

When the vegetables and meat are brown, add the liquids and the parsley to the pan and cover. Place the pan in the oven and roast for 3–4 hours, turning the meat every hour until tender.

Remove roast from the oven. Remove cover and let roast cool for about an hour.

When cooled, refrigerate until fat hardens. It is now easy to remove the fat. Slice roast and remove any fatty portions. The juices will have gelled. Heat juices just until liquefied. Process or blend the pot vegetables in the broth to thicken and produce delicious low-fat gravy.

Spoon the de-fatted gravy over the roast, cover with foil and heat in a 325° oven until warm. Arrange the roast on a serving platter and pour the gravy over the top.

*I've turned into the person I always
wanted to be.*

—Houstonian Kristin Vigeant,
who lost 90 pounds through exercise
and a sensible diet

Chapter 13

How Much Is Enough?

How much should you eat today? It's a tough question.

Back in chapter 5, you calculated approximately how many calories your body needs to meet your goals. In the chart below, we'll match those calorie counts to food.

Calories	Veggie Servings	Fruit Servings	Milk Servings	Meat	Starch Servings	Fat Servings
1,200	4+	2	1	5 oz.	6	3
1,400	4+	2	2	6 oz.	6	4
1,600	4+	2	2	7 oz.	7	5
1,800	4+	3	2	8 oz.	8	5
2,000	4+	3	3	9 oz.	8	6
2,200	4+	3	3	10 oz.	10	6
2,400	4+	4	3	12 oz.	10	7
2,600	4+	4	3	13 oz.	11	8
2,800	4+	4	4	13 oz.	12	9

If you didn't calculate your calorie intake in chapter 5, don't automatically drop to the bottom of this chart—most people don't need 2,800 calories a day. To lose weight, the average woman should consume 1,300 to 1,600 calories a day, and the average man 1,500 to 1,900. To maintain weight, the average woman needs 1,500 to 1,900, and the average man 1,900 to 2,400.

No one should ever try to consume less than 1,200 calories. At that point, you lower your metabolism. Your body puts itself in starvation mode and will work *not* to burn calories, in an effort to meet its survival needs. Less is not necessarily better.

This chart outlines quantity, but you must always remember quality as well. Not all starch or fat servings are created equal; a handful of pecans is far better for you than a handful of french fries. To keep your body strong, you must commit to the 80–20 rule, making the best-quality choices 80 percent of the time.

KEEPING TRACK

You will want to log your progress in both dietary improvements and exercise routines. Use a planner, appointment book, or notebook to monitor your work, assess your outcomes, and stay on track.

Are you wondering why everyone, regardless of their calorie count, is supposed to eat at least four vegetables a day—with no upper limit? It's simple: Because vegetables are low in calories and high in nutrients, you really can have as many as you like—in fact, the more, the better. (Just remember that starchy veggies count as starches, not vegetables.) Try to eat two servings of veggies at lunch every day, and two or more at dinner.

Once again: What's a serving?

It'll take you a little practice to answer that question. For a short time, while you're learning the ropes, you'll even have to measure things. But before you know it, you'll be able to visualize serving sizes without your measuring cups.

Below we provide a handy guide that you can copy and post on your refrigerator, or put in any other easily accessed spot in your kitchen.

To keep things simple, we've rounded off into half-cup or one-cup servings. Half a cup is about what will fit in one cupped hand (assuming yours aren't unusually big or small); one cup is about what will fit in both hands cupped together.

If you crave more precision, consider hiring a dietitian. Visit the American Dietetic Association Web site at www.eatright.org, or the American Diabetes Association Web site at www.diabetes.org.

Vegetables	1 cup raw veggies or salad
	½ cup cooked veggies (the size of a light bulb)
	6 oz. vegetable juice
Fruit	1 medium fruit (the size of a baseball)
	¾ cup sliced fruit
	½ cup cooked or canned fruit
	6 oz. 100 percent fruit juice (no more than one serving per day)
Milk	8 oz. milk or soymilk (small milk carton)
	6–8 oz. yogurt
	1.5 oz. cheese (the size of three dominoes)
	2 oz. processed cheese (American or Velveeta—the size of four dice)
Meat	2–3 oz. cooked meat, poultry, or fish
	(the size of a deck of cards or the palm of your hand)
	1 tbsp. peanut butter (the size of a ping-pong ball)
	1 egg or 2 egg whites
	¼ cup nuts
Starch	1 slice bread (if it has two sections—like an English muffin
	or bagel—count it as 2 servings)
	1 cup dry cereal (the size of a hockey puck)
	½ cup beans, corn, peas, or mashed potatoes
	½ cup cooked pasta, rice, or hot cereal (the size of half a baseball)
	6 wheat crackers
	3 cups no-fat popcorn
	12–15 reduced-fat chips
Fat	1 tsp. butter or oil (a pat the size of a stamp)
	1 tbsp. reduced-fat mayo (the size of your thumb tip)
	2 tbsp. reduced-fat salad dressing

Balancing your food checkbook

If you like, use the chart below to keep track of your daily intake. Make one copy, and use a marker to black out the boxes with numbers too high for your daily calorie needs. (For instance, if you need 1,400 calories a day, you need only two servings of fruit. So on the fruit line, you'd black out the boxes with numbers higher than two.)

Make copies of this personalized chart, and use one each day, checking off the servings as you eat them.

Your goal, of course, is to check off all the boxes you're allowed—and *at least* four vegetables, and *at least* eight glasses of water.

Daily Checklist

Category	Servings (or ounces of meat, or glasses of water)												
Veggie	1	2	3	4	5	6	7	8	9	10	11	12	13
Fruit	1	2	3	4	5	6	7	8	9	10	11	12	13
Milk	1	2	3	4	5	6	7	8	9	10	11	12	13
Meat	1	2	3	4	5	6	7	8	9	10	11	12	13
Starch	1	2	3	4	5	6	7	8	9	10	11	12	13
Fat	1	2	3	4	5	6	7	8	9	10	11	12	13
Water	1	2	3	4	5	6	7	8	9	10	11	12	13

Pizza Party!

Pizza can be so nutritious and fun for a crowd. Offering healthy ingredients and toppings, a build-your-own homemade pizza party is great entertainment for all ages.

Start with a pre-made crust, such as Boboli, or pre-bake one using your favorite recipe.

When slightly cooled, cut into squares and give each person their crust to embellish with toppings of their choice.

Toppings to offer:

Fresh tomatoes, seeded, sliced or diced
Fresh basil
Grated reduced-fat mozzarella cheese
Fresh bell peppers, seeded and sliced
Fresh mushrooms, sliced
Sliced olives
Bite-size pieces of cooked ham, chicken or steak
Fresh garlic, sliced or minced
Onion, sliced or chopped
Fresh jalapeños, seeded and sliced
Cubed pineapple
Zucchini
Asparagus
Sliced fennel
Broccoli
Celery
Spinach
Chard
Arugula

When your guests have their pizzas dressed, put them on a cookie sheet and bake at 350° until cheese is bubbly.

Grate a little fresh parmesan and enjoy.

Today the biggest decisions I make aren't
related to the heavyweight title.
They are whether I visit McDonald's,
Burger King, Wendy's or Jack-in-the-Box.

—George Foreman

Chapter 14

Cooking Better *and* Faster

So when, you wonder, are you going to find time to locate a recipe and cook something as exotic as quinoa? Your typical weeknight flies past in a blur. Getting any kind of dinner on the table feels like a burden, let alone a wholesome, nutrient-dense meal. You are tempted by the fast-food drive-through you pass on your way home. If nothing else, at least it's fast.

Resist that temptation. Do it for yourself: You know how bad that food is for your waistline. And do it for your family: The other adults will benefit from nutritious meals as much as you will, and your kids need good food even more, since they're learning the eating patterns that they'll carry with them for the rest of their life. It's estimated that 33 percent of U.S. children are overweight—no doubt in part because we've lost the habit of sitting down to dinner as a family.

Whatever your family situation—whether you have kids, you're single or married, working or retired—the following techniques will help you prepare healthy food faster. Yes, you'll have to commit at least a little time. Consider it an investment in your—and your family's—health.

- Bulk cooking once a week makes the most of your time in the kitchen. For instance, you might set aside some time every Sunday to prepare several foods that you can reheat throughout the week. With main dishes, consider cooking twice as much as your family will eat in the coming week—and freeze half for later meals.

- Do some of your prep work ahead of time. Immediately after returning home from the grocery store, wash all fruits and vegetables. Slice, chop and dice those you plan to grill, use in salads, and stir-fry. And be sure to have some ready to eat raw, displayed in a see-through container, for quick snacking.

- Prepare a large, fabulous salad with a good variety of veggies, and store it in an airtight container in your vegetable drawer. If it's a greens-based salad, do not add dressing or tomatoes until ready to serve, as the acid will cause the lettuce to wilt. Or instead of lettuce, try basing your salad on beans—black-eyed peas with chopped red and green peppers, tossed in a

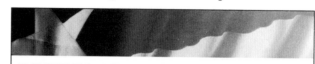

RECIPES AT LIGHT SPEED

Don't have time to riffle through your cookbooks? Use the Internet to look for recipes. Go to a search engine such as google.com and type in "low-fat quinoa recipe" or "tofu preparation" or "crock-pot beans"—whatever it is that you want. Or try these useful sites:

- www.epicurious.com
- www.foodfit.com
- www.mealsforyou.com
- www.nutritiouslygourmet.com
- www.cookinglight.com/cooking
- www.healthychoice.com

low-fat vinaigrette; chickpeas with loads of chopped parsley and other herbs, tossed in olive oil and vinegar and topped with low-fat feta; or black beans with tomatoes, onions, jalapeños, cilantro, olive oil, and lime juice. Those bean-based salads are not only nutritionally dense, they'll last beautifully in your fridge.

- Pack some or all of your lunches for the week ahead of time. If you put something in the fridge Sunday night, you can grab it easily on a hectic Tuesday morning—and you won't have to resort to fast food or vending-machine snacks.

- Organize your kitchen, starting with your pantry. (See chapter 10 for suggestions on stocking it.) Then move on to your kitchen drawers and cabinets. The better organized your work space, the more efficient you'll be.

- Keep a running grocery list, writing down items as you run out of them during the week.

- Be careful, in your quest for efficiency, not to lose sight of variety. Yes, it's easiest if breakfast is always the same, if the packed lunch never varies, and if dinner always consists of the same well-worn recipes. But such repetition can mean that you don't eat a wide variety of foods and so may be missing out on important nutrients.

   Besides, sameness can get awfully boring. Meals should be something you look forward to.

- Don't just throw your recipes into a drawer, where you'll have trouble finding them. Organize a notebook according to categories: meatless entrées, fish, poultry, meats, vegetables, breads, desserts, and so forth.

- Pull out the Crock-Pot. If you're not using it, you're missing out on a great way to cook long-simmered stews or flavorful pots of beans while you're not even in the house. If you don't already have one, look for a version with a removable center crock. At night, you can load it with your ingredients and stick it in the fridge. Then, in the harried morning, all you have to do is plop the crock into the heating unit and turn the dial to "cook." Dinner will be waiting for you when you get home.

What Texans can dream, Texans can do.

—George W. Bush

Chapter 15

How Much? How Soon?

Action Point Nine:
Set your goals

James L. Lundy, who lives in Wichita Falls, wrote these words:

If you don't know where you are going
... any path will get you there
... but you won't realize if you are lost
... you won't know what time you'll arrive
... you won't know the dimensions of your challenges
... others won't understand how they can help
... and since you could pass right by without recognizing it
... you won't get the satisfaction of having arrived!

Losing weight is like anything else you want to accomplish in life: It's important to have goals. For weight loss, the questions are, how much do you want to lose, and over what period of time?

So get out your pen and paper. It's time to write a contract with yourself. If you like, you can use the following model.

Goal Number One: My overall goal is to lose _____ pounds so that I weigh my healthy weight (as calculated in chapter 5), _____.

(If it seems too daunting to reach your healthy weight, remember that losing 10 percent of your current weight can bring many health benefits. Could you set a 10 percent weight loss as your initial goal?)

My target size for clothing is _____.

Goal Number Two: I will follow the Action Points for at least twelve months.

Goal Number Three: I will make adjustments to my plan if I reach a plateau and am not making further progress.

Goal Number Four: I believe steady weight loss is more effective than quick weight-loss programs, so I can accept a long-term goal of losing _____pounds within one year. The ending date is [twelve months from today].

MAKING IT HAPPEN

- Share your goals with your Texas Two-Step Partner.
- If you're a believer, ask God to help you set your goals.
- Make both short-term and long-term goals.
- Have both easy and difficult goals.
- Make your goals reasonable and believable.
- Make your health goals a high priority in your life.
- Put your goals in writing, and post them someplace highly visible. If they're easy to see, they'll be easy to keep in mind.
- You don't have to have deadlines for your goals as long as you're making progress.

My short-term weight goals are:

_____ pounds in_____ weeks

_____ pounds in_____ weeks

_____ pounds in_____ weeks

(These will be useful mileposts for measuring your progress. But remember that healthy weight loss is tricky, and that you may have to adjust your timetable.)

Goal Number Five: I will keep my weight under [your top healthy weight].

Consider these goals to be guideposts that will help you see how far you've traveled, and how far you have to go. Later in the journey, after you find that you're traveling faster or slower than you expected, you may want to adjust your goals. That's fine: They're _your_ goals.

Alternative to Action Point Nine

If you're not ready to set long-term goals, consider setting preliminary ones—say, a three-month goal instead of a one-year goal. Or get started with your plan first, and set your goals after you see how it's going.

I'm gonna spend my time
Like it's going out of style
I'm moving the bottom line
Farther than a country mile
I still have hills to climb
Before I hit that wall
No matter how much time I buy
I can never spend it all

—"Spend My Time,"
as sung by Clint Black

Chapter 16

Time to Reflect

Action Point Ten:
Make room in your schedule to stop and think

You can't lose weight and adopt great health habits over a weekend—not even a long weekend. If you're really going to change your life, you need to work on it a little every day.

To do that, you'll need to set aside some time each day to strengthen your dedication and determination. Start today. Tomorrow is another day, but that's no reason to waste today.

Every day you should:

- Set aside five to ten minutes to talk with your Two-Step Partner about your progress. (If your Two-Step Partner isn't available, journal your thoughts. Or pray.)
- Reread your letter to yourself—or at least remind yourself of the reasons you want to lose weight.
- Look at your Not Today List and remind yourself of the damage those foods inflict on your body. Remind yourself that today you will eat the right foods.
- Look at the list of your top five priorities. Ask yourself how you are going to spend time on them. Remember to spend time on first things first.
- Make this reflective time an important and inspirational part of your day.

Alternative to Action Point Ten

Create another daily list of activities that fits your personality and lifestyle better than the one above. Or follow the list above only on weekdays, or every other day. The point is to develop a regular routine to strengthen your resolve.

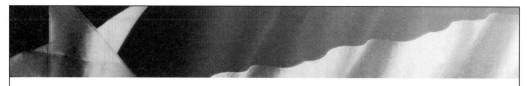

FINDING TIME

Where, you ask, can you find five to ten minutes in your day? Try skipping these things:

- One household chore that doesn't absolutely have to be done
- One TV show
- One video game
- One trip to the doughnut shop
- One beer after work
- One regular activity that doesn't contribute to your top five priorities

Or consider talking with your Two-Step Partner while you exercise.

Happy Hour

The downfalls of many are the after-work drinks that are full of calories and many that are not beneficial to our overall health and well-being. You can still have the occasional drink, but follow these tips to lighten up.

Wine or Champagne Spritzer

Add club soda to your wine or champagne for a lighter libation. For a White Wine Sangria, add fresh fruit (orange slices, berries and apples) as well as club soda to your wine. Adding ice to your wine glass will also boost your intake of water for the day while cooling off your drink.

Shandy

Add tart lemonade to your beer for a light, refreshing summer cooler.

Sancho Panza

Beer with tomato juice is great for a breakfast, brunch or hangover. (A little hair of the coyote that bit you.)

Rio Ruby

Enjoy your Ruby Red grapefruit juice with a several shakes of cayenne pepper, salt and a splash of club soda.

Texas Teresita

Add beef boullion and hot picante sauce to your tall glass of tomato juice over ice and finish off with a squeeze of fresh lime juice.

Hot peppers and picante lighten spirits and mood with fewer calories than alcohol. Skip the salted peanuts and chips and go for the healthy snacks mentioned on page 79.

Our being is subject to all the chances of life. There are so many things we are capable of, that we could be or do. The potentialities are so great that we never, any of us, are more than one-fourth fulfilled.

— Katherine Anne Porter

Chapter 17

Commitment

Action Point Eleven:
Commit to your success

Making a commitment to yourself is easy. The hard part, of course, is sticking with your commitment.

There are a number of ways to increase your chances of success:

1. Mean what you commit to, and commit to what you mean.
2. Make the commitment a part of your daily life. Discuss it with your Two-Step Partner, your spouse, and your friends. Pray about it. Think about it during your daily reflection time.
3. Follow all sixteen Action Points to success.
4. Put your commitment in writing as a contract with yourself. This is similar to the letter to yourself—only this time you're not explaining why you want to lose weight. You're promising yourself that you will. You can write your own contract or use the following:

> *This contract is to confirm my commitment to follow the sixteen Action Points in the* Texas Two-Step Diet. *I will perform these actions as described—and will make significant changes in my daily life.*

I will make good food choices, in terms of both quantity and quality, and will cheat very little. And I'll never cheat with the Not Today Foods I've promised myself to avoid.

I will exercise. I will check in every day with my Two-Step Partner. And I will take time each day to reflect on my accomplishments and challenges.

In all seriousness,
[Your name]
[Date]

Alternative to Action Point Eleven

You don't have to put your commitment in writing. But you *do* have to commit. The alternative—accepting failure before you even start—is lousy. Don't do that.

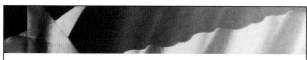

VIDEO INSPIRATION

If you feel yourself losing steam, rent a movie that shows what passionate commitment can accomplish.

Some good choices:

- *Breaking Away*
- *Erin Brockovich*
- *Field of Dreams*
- *Gandhi*
- *Hoosiers*
- *Lorenzo's Oil*
- *Million Dollar Baby*
- *Mr. Holland's Opus*
- *My Left Foot*
- *The Princess Bride*
- *Rain Man*
- *Rocky*
- *Schindler's List*
- *Seabiscuit*
- *Sense and Sensibility*
- *Shine*
- *The Sound of Music*
- *Spellbound*
- *Stand and Deliver*
- *Whale Rider*

The Thrill of the Grill

You can do your whole meal on the grill. Get the family out there with you—toss the baseball, pitch the horseshoes, play fetch with your dog, teach the children to swing a lariat and rope a stump.

Spice Rub for Meats

2 T. coarsely ground pepper
1 tsp. cumin
1 tsp. ground cayenne pepper
2 cloves garlic, finely minced
1 T. rosemary leaves, chopped

Combine and rub onto oiled (olive oil is best) meat. Allow meat to rest with rub on for a few minutes before cooking. Also a rub of just salt and pepper is delicious, too.

Use the Vinaigrette on page 37 as a marinade for squash, zucchini, onions, mushrooms, bell peppers and asparagus and grill them while you're grilling your meat.

Texas-Style Bruschetta

1 cup olive oil
1 jalapeño, seeded and finely chopped
2 T. cilantro, finely chopped
1 T. garlic, minced
Salt and pepper to taste
Whole-wheat bread

Mix well and let flavors combine. Brush this wonderful flavored olive oil onto bread and toast on the grill. Top with Salsa Fresca (see page 149).

You can also use the same process to make Texas Pita Toasts. Cut pita bread into wedges, brush with olive oil mixture and bake for 15 minutes at 300°—a yummy toasted 'cracker' for serving with Salsa Fresca.

I think Texans have more fun
than the rest of the world.

—Tommy Tune

Chapter 18

Just *Thinking* About Exercise

Action Point Twelve:
Get moving

You already know that you *should* exercise, that exercise is necessary to lose weight and stay healthy, and that it's good for your mental health. That's why, every six months or so, you lace up your walking shoes or check that schedule of yoga classes. But exercise doesn't work if it's sporadic. You have to stick with it.

Nike is wrong: You can't just do it. You have to make a long-term commitment. And you have to make it fun, so you can stick with that commitment.

To-do list:

1. If you aren't already exercising, commit to start right away.
2. Plan when and where you will exercise. Ask yourself what you'll enjoy doing. And figure out what you need to do it. Should you sign up for a class? Should you buy new gym clothes? Would it help to hire a personal trainer?
3. Get a logbook to record your exercise every day.

4. Consider working out with a friend or with your spouse. Odds are, he or she could use the exercise, too. You'll reinforce each other, and you'll both enjoy exercise more if you have company. It doesn't take two to Two-Step, but it's a lot more fun if you're not alone.

Just Moving

During a regular day, even when you're not in your cardio class or on the jogging trail, you move around—and that's good. The more you move, the more calories you burn.

It truly does make a difference to use the stairs instead of the elevator, to park farther from the building, and to deliver a message to a co-worker by walking to their desk versus e-mailing them. Any movement—even fidgeting—burns calories.

If you think about your day, you'll probably see easy ways to add more activity to your life. Could you commit never to park closer than a quarter-mile from your office building? Could you take the stairs from your office to the cafeteria and back each day? Are you walking your dog enough? (Exercise is good for pets, too.) And if you don't have a dog that needs walking, do you have a neighbor who'd appreciate your walking his pet?

A pedometer is a great cheap way to track your activity. You wear the inexpensive little device on your waistband, and it counts every step you take—whether you're training for a marathon or just walking to the water cooler. Most pedometers will have you measure your stride and set the device accordingly. Set it to match your typical daily stride, rather than your exercise stride, because that's how you move most of the day. Yes, it'll undercount your exercise steps, but not by much. And you'll know that, if anything, you actually took *more* steps that day.

Amy's clients tell encouraging stories about wearing pedometers. Just keeping track of your movement is inspiring. Some people set their computers to beep every 90 minutes, signaling that it's time for a five-minute walk break (about 200 steps on the pedometer). Some clients have even reported doing laps in the living room while on the phone, to try to increase their steps on days when they're falling short.

The first time you wear your pedometer, you'll want to get an idea of how many steps you take on an average day. Choose a day that seems likely to be typical, and wear your pedometer all day without looking at it.

You should aim, ultimately, to get in 10,000 steps every day—the equivalent of walking approximately five miles. It sounds like a lot, but of course you don't have to do all that walking at once.

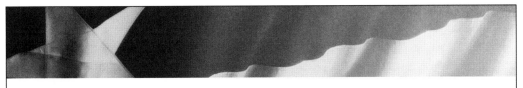

EXERCISE:
MAKING THE FIRST MOVE

- Do what you enjoy, and keep it simple.
- Incorporate variety. Cross-train to keep exercise interesting and to work different muscles.
- If you're getting bored, change the scenery. Try a new gym, park, walking path, or trail system.
- Look into activities sponsored by your Parks and Recreation Department.
- Always take the stairs.
- At work, park in the spot farthest from the door.
- Instead of e-mailing a co-worker, walk to deliver your message.
- Use the restrooms on a different floor at work—and take the stairs.
- Set your computer to sound an alarm every 90 minutes. When it beeps, it's time for you to take a short walk break.
- Vacuum the house with vigor.
- Do yard work or putter in the garden.
- Don't use the remote control.
- Go dancing.
- If you're not exercising at all, start by scheduling your exercise time every Sunday evening. Write it in your appointment book, and treat it as something not to be missed!
- Wash your own car.
- Park as far from your destination as the parking lot permits.
- Fly a kite.

To build up to 10,000 steps, start at your baseline, and aim to take 2,000 more steps each day. For instance, if your baseline is 3,000 steps, aim for 5,000. After you've done that successfully for two weeks, bump up your goal by another 2,000 steps for another two weeks. Eventually, you'll hit 10,000 steps.

Alternative to Action Point Twelve

You *must* get moving. But if exercise seems intimidating, start by simply working more activity into your daily life.

Quickie Smoothie

This vitamin-packed smoothie is great not only for breakfast, but also serves as a great after-workout energy boost. Kids love it, and you get much of your recommended daily fruit servings in one blast!

Combine in blender:
1 cup nonfat yogurt
1 banana, sliced (If you have over-ripe bananas, peel, slice and freeze—these make a frostier smoothie)
¼ cup orange juice
1 cup of your favorite fruit or combination:
   Berries, peaches, pears, plums, grapes, mango or pineapple

---

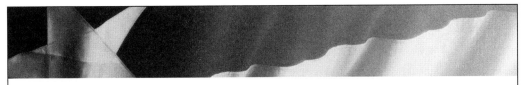

EXERCISE:
MAKING THE FIRST MOVE

- Throw a Frisbee with a friend.
- Join an organization to help clean up your community.
- Walk to the grocery store for small purchases.
- Walk the entire mall and window-shop before going into a store.
- Limit your television and computer time.
- Do calf-raises in the shower.
- Plan a family outing that includes physical activity. Hikes, bike rides, and walks are great.
- See the sights by walking.
- When golfing, walk the course rather than using a cart.
- Play singles tennis or racquetball instead of doubles.
- During picnics, play volleyball or badminton rather than horseshoes.
- Get off the bus or train a few blocks early.
- Take a brisk walk when you have the urge to snack.
- Stay at hotels with fitness centers.
- Walk while waiting for your plane.
- Brainstorm projects with co-workers while on a walk rather than at a desk.
- Stand up and pace while on the phone.
- Walk around the house during commercials.
- Make homemade bread, kneading the dough by hand.
- Rent an exercise video instead of a movie.
- Do household chores while the TV is on.

Plan the work and work the plan.

—Charles T. Bridgman,

John Bridgman's dad

Chapter 19

Progress Report

Action Point Thirteen:
Measure your progress

Business consultants often say, "What gets measured and rewarded gets done." And they're right. Just recording the data forces you to pay attention and lets you know how you're doing. Everyone wants to see good reports.

So get yourself a notebook, and dedicate one page to each day's results. Each day, you should:

- In your log book, record exactly what you had for breakfast, lunch and dinner. Use the chart from chapter 13 if you like.
- Record any snacks and when you ate them.
- List what you had to drink throughout the day.
- Record any exercise.
- List ways you tried to get in additional activity. Did you walk the dog? Take the stairs at work?
- Ask yourself, did you have any foods from your Not Today List? If so, what can you do to prevent yourself from making the same mistake tomorrow?
- Ask yourself, did you have to deal with emotional eating situations? How did your plan work?

- Record your weight once a week. Always use the same scale, and weigh yourself at approximately the same time each day.
- Last, ask yourself, how did you feel about your day? How did you do?

Then, use your notebook to plan your day.
- What do you plan to do differently today with meals and snacks?
- What can you can look forward to doing today?
- How will you focus on your priorities?
- What can you do for someone else today?
- When will you get in your exercise?

Alternative to Action Point Thirteen

Measure your progress every other day instead of every day. Or focus on your eating and exercise.

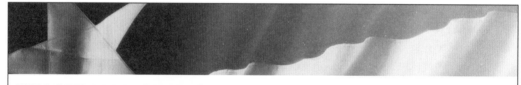

MEASURABLE SUCCESS

- When you complete your daily to-do list, take a moment to congratulate yourself.
- Plan to be considerate today, tomorrow and always.
- Today eliminate two or three things that are a waste of time. And eliminate them for good.
- Instead of watching TV, do something productive. Or at least do something productive *while* watching TV. Knit. Cook. Jog in place. Do sit-ups. You get the idea.
- Take advantage of today to make good things happen.

Make it fun!

Dieting and exercising do not have to be a drag. Include your family in the gardening—children are great at weeding and planting seeds.

Cooking together really can bring a family together. Give everyone a job: cutting out jicama stars, setting the table, toasting the nuts, washing the vegetables, cutting the herbs—there is a job for any age.

Try chili and everyone can add their favorite toppings—low-fat cheese, chopped onions, nonfat sour cream, jalapeños, cilantro....

Try curry with extra sambals or toppings—cucumber, chopped eggs, mango, onion, mushrooms, cashews, peanuts....

Have a family salad bar—offer various lettuce types (iceberg, romaine, Boston, spinach); let everyone have a choice of toppings: beets, artichokes, asparagus, corn, peas, beans, cottage cheese, sliced apple, sliced orange, berries, snow peas, cucumbers, peppers (fresh or roasted), carrots, tomatoes, chopped ham, chicken, turkey or steak. The list can go on and on....

Make a healthy sundae—use frozen nonfat yogurt with these healthy topping choices: mango, berries, peaches, nectarines, bananas, nuts, low-fat granola....

I don't need to ride for the money.
I would happily ride for nothing.
I will be riding a bike in ten years' time
because I feel better when I do exercise
and I want to enjoy true good health.

—Lance Armstrong

Chapter 20

Sweating

Action Point Fourteen:
Commit to a real exercise program

I f you simply cut calories to lose weight, you'd lose a little of everything that makes up your body: some fat, some water, and some muscle. But, of course, you don't *want* to lose muscle, because muscle burns calories. That's why it's important to exercise.

You should aim to get in both cardiovascular activity (the kind that raises your heart rate) and resistance training (the kind that builds muscle).

The American College of Sports Medicine and the U.S. Centers for Disease Control and Prevention have found that 30 minutes of moderate-intensity exercise, performed most days of the week, will improve your health. The longer and harder you work, the greater the health benefits will be. To lose weight, or to avoid losing muscle as you age, you should aim for 60 minutes of cardiovascular activity most days of the week.

That seems like a lot. But you can get there.

Aerobic Exercise

Aerobic exercise is any kind of movement that gets your heart pumping faster and keeps it pumping for a while. But how fast should your heart pump? Here's a formula.

1. To calculate your maximum heart rate, subtract your age from 220.

   • For example, if you're 35, the math would be:
     220–35=185
     Therefore, your maximum heart rate would be 185.

2. You want to exercise at 70 to 85 percent of your maximum heart rate. To get that range, multiply your maximum heart rate by .7, and then by .85.

   • For the person above, 70 percent would be:
     185 × 0.7=129.5
     and 85 percent would be:
     185 × 0.85=157.2
   So this person should aim to exercise so that his heart rate falls between 130 and 157 beats per minute, a rate at which he's breathing noticeably harder than usual, but can still talk easily.

Here are some kinds of exercise likely to help you hit your target heart rate:

- Aerobics (step, kickboxing, low-impact, water aerobics, etc.)
- Basketball
- Biking (outdoors or on a stationary bike)
- Boxing
- Circuit training
- Cross-country skiing
- Dancing vigorously
- Elliptical machine
- Hockey
- Jumping rope
- Jumping on a trampoline

- Kayaking
- Racquetball
- Rock climbing
- Rollerblading
- Running/jogging (outdoors or on a treadmill)
- Rowing
- Rugby
- Skateboarding
- Spinning class
- Squash
- Stairs (real ones or a StairMaster)
- Swimming
- Tennis
- Walking briskly

Aerobic Exercise for Absolute Beginners

If you're like most Texans, and haven't been exercising at all, it's a good idea to consult your doctor before you begin—especially if you're over 40, are pregnant, have had heart trouble or diabetes, or are taking medication for any chronic condition.

- Begin slowly. Start with three ten-minute sessions of cardiovascular exercise a day, three times a week. Stay at that level for two weeks.
- Then build up to two fifteen-minute sessions a day, three times a week. And stay at that level for two weeks.
- Now you're ready for thirty-minute sessions, three times a week. Congratulations! Consider that the absolute minimum for good health.
- But the minimum, of course, isn't what you're aiming for. You want to lose weight and retain muscle mass as you age. You don't want to feel good, you want to feel *great*. Start working out four times a week for thirty minutes. And do that for two weeks.
- Then increase to five times a week; continue to increase every two weeks until you are exercising six times a week for thirty minutes.

Building Endurance

For some people, aerobic exercise six times a week for 30 minutes is not enough to lose weight or even to maintain a healthy weight. If this is the case for you, you'll want to increase the number of minutes you're exercising each day. And once again, you'll want to build up slowly.

- Start by working out for thirty minutes five days a week, and forty-five minutes one day a week. Continue for two weeks.
- Work out for thirty minutes four days a week, and for forty-five minutes two days a week. Continue for two weeks.
- Keep adding one longer session every two weeks until you're exercising for forty-five minutes a day, six days a week.
- Then increase one of your workouts to 60 minutes.
- After two weeks, increase another of your weekly workouts to 60 minutes.
- Continue until you are working out for 60 minutes a day, six days a week.

Variety

Variety is as important with exercise as it is with food. It adds interest. A change of pace will make your workout feel like play time—and if exercise is fun, you'll have an easier time sticking with it.

But changing your routine is also good for your body. If you're a runner, your body becomes efficient at running. But running doesn't use the same muscles that biking uses. And biking doesn't use the same muscles that rowing or swimming or aerobics class uses. The more different things you do, the better balanced your body will be.

Aim to incorporate at least three cardiovascular activities into your life. Most likely, you'll have a favorite activity, which will be your top choice the majority of the time. But make sure that every week you are doing at least two activities, and most weeks you have done each of the three activities at least once.

The Power of Intervals

Once you're exercising three times a week at your target heart rate, it's time to put interval training in your exercise program.

Interval training adds short bursts of high-intensity work to your regular workout. For instance, if you're a jogger, you'd jog at your regular pace, then sprint for a while, then return to your regular pace. Those bursts force your body to work differently, and are often very beneficial in helping those who hit a plateau with either their weight-loss efforts or their level of endurance.

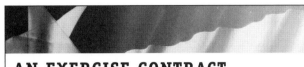

AN EXERCISE CONTRACT

Try putting your exercise commitment in writing with a contract like this one:

For the next two weeks, I commit to _____ days a week of cardiovascular exercise and _____ days a week of resistance training. And after that, I intend to build my workouts as outlined in the *Texas Two-Step Diet*.

- Begin by adding three one-minute intervals to your workout twice a week. Sustain this for the first two weeks.
- Then increase to five one-minute intervals twice a week, for two consecutive weeks.
- Now change to three two-minute intervals, twice a week.
- Increase to five two-minute intervals, twice a week.
- Over time you can build to five two-minute intervals three times a week. There is no need to go over this level.

Some examples of intervals include:

- Walking at your target heart rate, and adding an interval by increasing your pace or incorporating a hill.
- Biking at your target heart rate, and adding intervals by moving into a standing position or incorporating hills.
- When jogging at your target heart rate, add intervals by sprinting a certain number of blocks, or to landmarks such as a house or lamppost.

Strength Training

Cardio alone isn't enough. You also need strength training to improve bone mass and build muscle and connective tissue. Strength training usually involves equipment that builds muscle, and it's essential to improving your body composition by increasing your lean body mass. The more muscle you have, the more calories you'll burn even while you're sleeping or working in front of a computer. What more could you ask?

No, you don't have to join a gym—though that's certainly a good option. Many pieces of strength-training equipment are modestly priced and can be used in your own home. But proper technique is essential, so try to work with a personal trainer, if only for the few sessions that it takes you to learn the correct way to work out.

Your strength-training workouts should challenge your muscles, improve your flexibility, and incorporate a mind-body element. Here are some of the pieces of equipment you might use:

- Weight machines
- Free weights
- Dumbbells
- Barbells
- Resistance tubes
- Bands
- Core boards
- Resist-A-Balls
- Medicine balls

Intensity

Each time you perform a movement, such as lifting a barbell, it's called a repetition, or "rep." You should choose the heaviest weight at which you can perform two sets of ten to fifteen reps. For instance, if you are performing bicep curls with ten-pound dumbbells, but can perform only six reps on your second set, then that weight is too heavy; you should drop down to eight-pound weights. Once you can complete two sets of reps, stay at that weight for two weeks, then move up to the next weight option, instead of adding another set or adding more reps to each set. The best way to gain strength is to make the muscle work harder, not longer.

Frequency

Current research recommends strength training two to three times a week on most weeks. When you are able to commit to twice a week, you will reap the most benefit by doing full-body workouts that build both your upper and lower body. If you're working out three times a week, you could either do full-body workouts or spend one day targeting your upper body, one day targeting your lower body, and one day working your whole body. Always be sure to work the larger muscles first, and start with your most difficult exercises. For instance, if push-ups and squats are difficult for you, do them at the beginning of your workout—not at the end, when you're tired.

Duration

You can build muscle and reduce fat with twenty to thirty minutes of quick-paced exercise, with no more than thirty seconds to one minute between exercises.

Genes

Your genetic makeup will determine the effect of strength training on your body. The most obvious gene, of course, is your sex chromosome. Amy's female clients commonly say that they avoid strength training because they fear they'll develop muscles like Arnold Schwarzenegger's. They needn't worry: Women don't put on muscle like that. And a lean, muscular female body is attractive. Just think about the women you've seen in the Olympics. Those pretty volleyball and tennis players lift weights several times a week.

But your body has other genes, too. Both men and women are born as one of three body types, each of which puts on muscle in a different way.

- **Mesomorphs** have muscular or stockier builds, and they build muscle faster than the other body types.
- **Endomorphs** tend to be round and voluptuous. They typically have to lose body fat to see changes in their shape.
- **Ectomorphs** are long, slender and lean. They tend to gain strength but don't build as much muscle as the other body types. Most women long to be ectomorphs, but only 10 percent of the population is born one.

Functional Exercise

Have you ever felt like you were in good shape, but threw your back out when you lifted a sixty-pound suitcase into the trunk of your car? You may be toned, but are you ready to hoist that spring-water bottle onto the dispenser?

Conventional weight training focuses on the largest muscles. No weight routine will train every muscle in your body or teach your muscle groups to work together. That's where functional fitness comes in.

Functional fitness focuses on building a body that is capable of doing real-life activities in real-life positions. The first step is often learning to balance your body and lift your own weight. Start with simple movements like one-legged squats and other balancing exercises. Then try standing on one leg on a step stool, approximately eight inches off the ground. Slowly bend your leg, lowering your free foot to the ground, then stand slowly back up, controlling your body weight as you go. After you've done that a few times, switch legs.

Once you are able to balance you own body weight, you can add weights to the exercises. Or try using other tools, such as stability balls, core boards or wobble boards—all of which force you to maintain your balance.

Incorporating functional exercise into everyday activities can be done easily. Try doing push-ups with hands on the kitchen counter while cooking or try lifting grocery bags to the sides and front of the body while unloading groceries from the car. Do calf raises in the shower or at the vanity in the morning or tricep dips on a chair or ottoman. Also try picking up a heavy bag of laundry: with feet square and shoulder width apart, squat and pick up the bag, pushing up with your legs. Set the bag back down and repeat.

You can't do functional exercise with the same intensity as regular weight lifting. If you train to failure (muscle fatigue), you train to fail. Instead, your set ends when you can no longer perform the exercise with perfect form.

Join Me for a Cup of Tea?

Herbal teas are full of antioxidants and stress relievers. When you add your own fresh herbs, they are injected with fresh wonderful flavors.

Herbal Tea

Use any of these herbs for a soothing drink anytime:

Ginger
Rosemary
Licorice
Chamomile
Orange
Tangerine
Lemon
Lemon Balm
Mint

For 1 cup, use approximately 1 T. fresh herbs
For 1 pot, use a handful of fresh herbs
Boil water; drop in herb (with regular tea bag, if desired) for 4 minutes or longer if you like a stronger brew.

Flavored Water

Can you really ever get too much water? Here's another way to enjoy it.
Instead of buying expensive flavored bottled water, make your own. This is pretty to look at as well as to drink … and great for parties and kids.

In a large pitcher, combine:
Water
Any combination of sliced oranges, lemons, limes, apples, strawberries, peaches
And a few sprigs of mint or lemon balm

You can have anything in this world you want, if you want it badly enough and you're willing to pay the price.

—Mary Kay Ash

Chapter 21

Temptation

Action Point Fifteen:
Tackle temptation

By now, you know good and well which foods will lead you into obesity. You know that a little of anything is okay—but what about when you're tempted to break the 80–20 rule and eat a whole carton of Blue Bell? What do you do when that gorgeous pecan pie calls your name? How will you handle all-you-can-eat buffets with fried chicken and barbecued ribs?

The key to tackling temptation is to have a clear conscience with the confidence, certainty and courage to be successful. Those four Cs will give you the strength to resist even cheese enchiladas—or, at least, to eat just one.

Conscience means that you know that by losing weight, you're doing the right thing for the right reasons.

Confidence means that you know you're strong enough to reach your goals. And it helps that your Two-Step Partner believes in you, too.

Certainty that you'll succeed makes it fun to tackle temptation. Look at each temptation as being amusing or harmless. Of course you can vanquish a peach cobbler, or withstand the siren call of a double-decker chili cheeseburger. You are the master of your own destiny. You will fear no french fry.

Courage makes you brave enough to resist that french fry, even when your conscience, confidence and certainty waver.

When you're facing temptation, offer yourself an alternative. Wouldn't you rather take a walk than eat all your kids' Halloween candy? Wouldn't a bowl of luscious Hill Country peaches end the meal as well as double-fudge cake? And shouldn't you have a glass of water or unsweetened tea instead of a Frappuccino?

It might help, too, to imagine how you'll feel an hour or two *after* you've resisted. If you successfully pass up one of the Not Today Foods that you've promised yourself to avoid, you'll feel good about yourself. But if

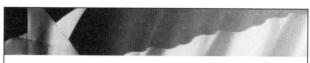

SAYING NO

When temptation beckons, try the following phrases:

"It isn't important!"

"It doesn't matter!"

"I don't need it."

"I know what those extra calories will do to my body."

"I can resist it, and I will beat it."

"This temptation will pass quickly, and I can outlast it."

"I've made a commitment to myself."

"I could use some fresh air."

"I think I'll have a glass of water instead."

you've devoured a whole bag of potato chips, you'll feel guilty, weak—and heavy.

Think about it: Feel good by tackling the temptation, or feel guilty by cheating on yourself. It's your call!

Alternative to Action Point Fifteen

If you're not up to facing temptation head-on, at least go out of your way to avoid it. Can't resist ribs? Don't eat at a barbecue joint. Do you feel politeness requires you to eat birthday cake? Make a polite excuse and skip the party.

Get Your Just Desserts!

It's just not fair to never have dessert. This sauce includes vitamin-rich fruits and can be served alone, over angel food cake, with biscotti, over nonfat sorbet or with ginger snaps.

Fruit with Wine Sauce

3 cups wine (whatever you have, but include some red because it makes a nice
    color for your sauce)
1 cup sugar, or ½ cup sugar and ¼ cup Splenda
6 cinnamon sticks
2 T. whole cloves
Zest or grated peel from 2 oranges and or 3 lemons

Cook wine mixture slowly for 2 hours.

Here's where the fruit comes in—add these to your Wine Sauce.

Choose your favorite, experiment with the flavors …
• Pears—Poach whole pears until barely tender; poach sliced pears for 5 minutes
• Apples—Poach sliced apples for 5 minutes
• Peaches—Slice in a bowl and pour warm sauce over to cover
• Berries—Same as peaches
• Oranges—Same as peaches
• Mango—Same as peaches
• Pineapple—Same as peaches

Serve fruit in shallow bowls with a cooked cinnamon stick and a little sauce.

The here and now is all we have,
and if we play it right, it's all we'll need.

—Former governor Ann Richards

Chapter 22

Fiesta Time

Action Point Sixteen:
Celebrate your success

Yes! It's time to pat yourself on the back!

There are many ways to celebrate your success. And yes, it's important that you *do* celebrate: Making a big deal of your accomplishments reinforces your determination.

And besides, it's just plain fun.

Right now, sit down and make yourself one last set of lists. Write "Celebrating" at the top of the page. Then think of at least one concrete way that you can do each of these things.

- Start the morning by choosing something to look forward to during the day.
- Do something creative. Write! Draw! Build! Knit! Design a Web site! Cook a healthy meal!
- Do something that reinforces your other priorities. Plan an outing with your kids. Meet a friend for a fruit smoothie.
- Perform a little act of kindness. Leave a huge tip. Let a tired mom cut in line. Mow your neighbor's yard. Send flowers, just because.
- Devote time to yourself. What is it that you'd really, really love to do?
- Buy yourself a great new outfit in your new size.

- Throw a party to celebrate your weight loss. Serve healthy food: sparkling water with lemon twists, grilled salmon, wild rice, spinach sautéed with garlic, and fruit salad. And wear your great new outfit.

Alternative to Action Point Sixteen

Okay, fine. Make yourself miserable. But remember, it wasn't our idea.

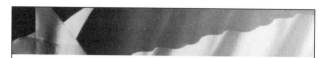

REASONS TO CELEBRATE

- Celebrate your faith and what it means to you.
- Celebrate what brings happiness to you and others.
- Celebrate your life and your health.
- Celebrate the differences, challenges, opportunities, and choices in life.
- Stop worrying about the traffic. Celebrate the journey and the destination.

Mexican Fiesta, Olé!

Salsa Fresca

Use what you have in your garden or refrigerator. Start with tomatoes, onions, lime juice and jalapeños, then add cilantro, bell peppers, mangos, pineapple, garlic, and chilies. Add a little salt and pepper to taste. Serve with Baked Tortilla Chips (see page 79).

Guacamole

Avocados are relatively high in calories, but are laden with vitamins. For health-conscious Guacamole, blend in other stretching vegetables. Mash an avocado with a fork, add chopped onions, tomatoes, lettuce, and jalapeños; a squeeze of lemon juice and salt and pepper to taste. Serve with Baked Tortilla Chips.

For an even lighter guacamole and further reduction of fat, use equal amounts of mashed, uncooked frozen green peas to stretch the avocado.

Grilled Fajitas

1½–2 pounds lean skirt steak or flank steak
½ cup fresh lime or lemon juice
4 cloves garlic, minced
½ onion, chopped
2 T. olive oil
1 tsp. salt
2 large sweet Texas onions, sliced into ½-inch thick rounds
Poblano, bell, jalapeño or your favorite type of pepper

Marinate the steak for 1–3 hours as time permits.

Grill the steak, onion slices and peppers, over a hot charcoal and mesquite fire 4–5 minutes per side or until desired doneness is reached. Remove to a platter or cutting board and allow to rest for 5 minutes before slicing thinly, across the grain. Serve immediately with grilled onions and peppers. Serves 4–6.

Black Beans

1 pound dry black beans
Basic Chicken Broth (see page 25)
1 clove garlic, minced
1 small onion, minced
Cilantro

Soak beans overnight if time permits. Drain and rinse and put into pot and cover with Basic Chicken Broth. Bring to boil, reduce heat and simmer one hour. Add more liquid throughout the cooking time to keep beans covered.

Add garlic and onion and simmer 1–1½ hours, or until beans are tender.

Add cilantro and serve. Serves 6–8.

Mexican Brown Rice

1 T. olive oil
1 medium onion, chopped
2 carrots, peeled and chopped
3 stalks celery, chopped
1 cup brown rice
2 cups chicken broth
1 cup water
½ tsp. salt
1–2 jalapeño peppers, seeded and chopped
1 T. chopped fresh parsley
1 T. chopped fresh cilantro

Heat oil in a heavy saucepan with a tight-fitting lid or Dutch oven, then add the onion, carrot, and celery. Sauté quickly for a couple minutes but do not brown. Add the rice, broth, water and salt, and bring to a boil. Cover and simmer over low heat for 45 minutes, or until rice is tender. Add the chopped pepper, parsley and cilantro. Replace cover and let stand for 5–10 minutes. Serve while hot … fragrant and steaming. Serves 4–6.

Gazpacho

A wonderful lunch made with fresh summer tomatoes.

4–6 fresh tomatoes, seeded and quartered
1 cucumber, halved lengthwise and seeded
4 spring onions with 2–3 inches of tender green tops, sliced
2 T. chopped Texas sweet onion
1 clove garlic, minced (optional)
1 jalapeño, seeded and chopped (optional)
2–3 sprigs parsley and/or cilantro
1 cup V-8 juice or tomato juice or water
2 T. vinegar
2 T. olive oil
Salt and pepper to taste

Pulse vegetables and herbs in a food processor or blender until chopped but not puréed … leave a little texture. Add tomato juice, vinegar, oil, salt and pepper. Serve with Texas Pita Toasts (see page 121) for a cool and satisfying summer lunch.

For a cold-weather pick-me-up, enjoy a cup of virtually no-calorie, no-fat hot bouillon (beef, chicken or vegetable). Add a few of your favorite chopped herbs and season to taste.

The Action Points

One: Sit right down and write yourself a letter.

Two: Figure out what's important.

Three: Ask for help.

Four: Analyze yourself.

Five: Make your shopping list.

Six: Recognize your trigger points—and hold your fire.

Seven: Stock your pantry.

Eight: Get rid of the bad, and don't overdo the good stuff.

Nine: Set your goals.

Ten: Make room in your schedule to stop and think.

Eleven: Commit to your success.

Twelve: Get moving.

Thirteen: Commit to a real exercise program.

Fourteen: Measure your progress.

Fifteen: Tackle temptation.

Sixteen: Celebrate your success.